Sports, Everyone!

Recreation and Sports for the Physically Challenged of All Ages

THE
LILIAN S. BESORE
MEMORIAL LIBRARY
GREENCASTLE, PENNSYLVANIA
FOUNDED MARCH 20, 1963

CONWAY GREENE PUBLISHING COMPANY

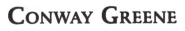

Other books from Conway Greene:

Athletic Scholarships: A Complete Guide
ISBN 1-884669-05-0

Art & Design Scholarships: A Complete Guide
ISBN 1-884669-06-9

Music, Dance & Theater Scholarships: A Complete Guide
ISBN: 1-884669-07-7

National Service Corps: A State-by-State Guide
ISBN 1-884669-03-4

School-to-Work Programs: A State-by-State Guide
ISBN 1-884669-04-2

Americorps: Serve Your Country and Pay for College
ISBN1-884669-12-3

Contents

Preface

The idea for *Sports, Everyone!* grew out of the research we did for our publication, *Athletic Scholarships: A Complete Guide* (1994). In that book, we researched several wheelchair sports scholarships. During that process we heard comments from athletic directors and coaches regarding equity issues for wheelchair athletes and other recreation opportunities for the physically challenged. We decided to pursue this topic in order to bring together recreation and sports resources which would be of interest to the physically challenged of all ages: from camps and playgrounds through college and on, into community activities, organized sports, travel and tourism, the ADA, and technology.

The focus of the book is *participation*, from the novice participant to the elite olympian. To learn how to participate in different sports, we have provided national organization information, with local and chapter contacts where available. A sport and activity index will help the reader find relevant organizations. ADA and Assistive Technology project information is provided at the state level. Colleges with premier programs for the physically challenged are covered along with the colleges which participate in the Wheelchair Basketball Central Intercollegiate Conference. In addition, the full Wheelchair Basketball roster is provided. Camps with programs for the physically challenged are listed with contact and cost information in addition to description of facilities and "camperships." Travel information is provided from the Department of the Interior as well as from individual parks and attractions.

We have also provided a planner by special recreation expert John A. Nesbitt, Professor Emeritus of the University of Iowa, who insisted we broaden the scope of this book to special recreation, which provides many outlets for creative and healthy activity beyond organized sports. This planner should be of help to anyone who is trying to incorporate recreation activities into his or her schedule. The planner will help the user think of new activities, understand the costs and barriers, and provide a framework for organizing an enhanced calendar.

We are particularly proud to offer the compelling life story of Jean Driscoll, competitive athlete and coach at the University of Illinois. At the time she originally wrote this article for this book she had won five Boston Marathons and was training for number six, which she went on to win. After you read her story, you will see that her marathon victories are not the only measures of her great success.

The publisher would like to thank the following people who contributed material, ideas, or other assistance to this publication:

Jim Angelo, Paralyzed Veterans Association

Kirk M. Bauer, Executive Director, Disabled Sports, USA

Shirley Boltz, Public Relations Manager of the American Camping Association

Jim Coombes, Executive Director, National Amputee Golf Association

Jean Driscoll, Athlete and Coach

Shad Dahlgren, Wheelchair Athlete

Jennifer Hester, USABA

John A. Nesbitt, President, Special Education, Inc.

Ron Tucker, Database Manager of Ohio T.R.A.I.N.

The Publisher would also like to thank Pat Phillips, Editor, and Lisa Hansen, Editorial Assistant, for their work compiling and editing the book and Mario Cavlovicak, Phoenix Promotion and Publishing, for the cover illustration.

The Publisher
Spring 1995

Introduction

The challenges in special recreation for the 43 million Americans who are disabled are enormous:

Among the millions of children, youth, adult, and senior Americans who are disabled, only two in ten are receiving optimal special recreation services; eight of ten are underserved or unserved.

65% of adults who are disabled are unemployed and live a depressed recreation lifestyle. They are not receiving the special recreation services they need.

75% of the millions of children and youth in special education schools and programs today are tracking to unemployment and a depressed recreation lifestyle. Special education is not providing these students the recreation education they need.

People who are disabled are underrepresented in public (tax supported) arts, culture, museums, parks and recreation, outdoor recreation, and sport activities at the local, state, and national level.

Among Americans who are disabled, 95% have little awareness of the vast development in special recreation that has occurred since the 1950s. That 95% is not aware of the recreation opportunities that are available and, therefore, do not seek opportunities for recreation.

Special recreation is important for so many reasons—affective, cognitive, developmental, emotional, health, physical, social, spiritual, and therapeutic. It is part of the pursuit of happiness fundamental to American life.

Sports, Everyone! Recreation and Sports for the Physically Challenged of All Ages addresses the need for information. *Sports, Everyone!* is a major step forward in providing access to the "American Recreation Lifestyle"—for everyone.

John A. Nesbitt, Ed.D.
President, Special Recreation, Inc. and
Director of the International Center on
Special Recreation
Professor Emeritus, University of Iowa

Just Rolling Along

by Jean Driscoll
Assistant Coach, Wheelchair Track & Field, University of Illinois

*Note: On April 17, 1995, Olympic Silver Medalist Jean Driscoll won
her sixth consecutive Boston Marathon.*

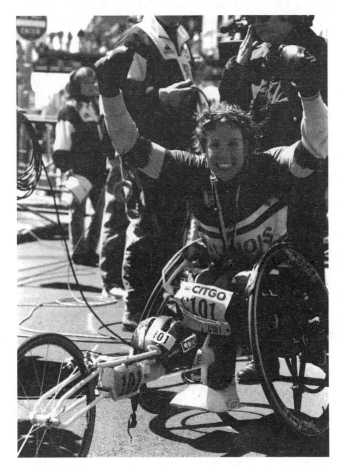

*Jean Driscoll after
winning her sixth Bos-
ton Marathon (Photo
courtesy PVA/Sports
'n Spokes/Curt
Beamer)*

All things considered, I've had a pretty amazing life. Although I
was born with spina bifida (an opening in the spine), I've had life experiences about which many people can only dream. For example, I have
won the Boston Marathon five times and have set a new world record
every time I've competed in it. I own an Olympic silver medal from the
1992 Olympic Games in Barcelona, Spain. During my time as a collegiate wheelchair basketball player, I had the opportunity of playing on
two national championship teams.

Aside from athletics, I have also had success in the classroom. I earned an undergraduate degree in Speech Communication and graduated with honors. I continued my education and also earned a master's degree in Rehabilitation Administration. As an undergraduate student, I received several accolades such as the University of Illinois Dad's Association's Outstanding Student of the Year. I was chosen out of 36,000 students for this award. Additionally, I received the prestigious Lincoln Student Laureate Award. This honor is presented by the governor at the state capitol and given to students who exemplify proficiency both inside and outside the classroom. Again, out of 30,000 students on campus, I was chosen. (All of this after flunking out of school a few years earlier!)

The success I've enjoyed has been the result of a lot of hard work. I have neither failed nor succeeded because of my disability. I have failed and succeeded because of my ability; that's the way life works. One tenet I live my life by is that you have to experience failure in order to appreciate success. People who are successful are not born that way. They are the ones who "get back on the horse every time they fall off." They accept setbacks as a way of learning and becoming stronger. If I ever write a book, I'm going to entitle it, "Still Falling Off the Horse."

I don't think it's a secret that a disability can be a setback. As a child, I experienced many setbacks. I never understood my disability. I didn't understand why I needed braces to walk, why my muscles were so much weaker than my sister's and brothers', why I couldn't run as fast as the other kids, and even more humiliating, why I couldn't control my bowel and bladder function like everyone else.

My self-esteem was low. I wanted to be a star athlete like the popular kids in school, yet, I scarcely could participate in sport at all. I could hit the softball, but I couldn't get to base fast enough.

I could throw the basketball up at the basket, but I couldn't run back and forth down the court. I could serve the volleyball, but I didn't have the balance to stand there and volley it over the net like the other kids. Adapted athletics? Never heard of it! I went to a grade school where I was the only person with a disability.

Fortunately I did have one thing in my life I could control and I got a lot of satisfaction from it, too. School. I wasn't a straight "A" student but I was usually among the students who got higher marks in class. It was the one area where I could compete with the other kids and not be last. Although doing homework was less fun than going outside to play or watching TV, I liked to reap the benefits of getting all my work done and doing well on tests.

Upon entering high school, my life took a dramatic change. About 2-1/2 months into my freshman year of high school, I had a bike accident. I was riding a ten-speed bike that I had won the previous year for reading the most books and raising the most money in a Read-a-Thon sponsored by the Multiple Sclerosis Society. I was going around a corner and took it too sharp. My left pedal caught the pavement and I slammed down on my hip. I dislocated it. I laid there about five or ten minutes and by the grace of God, my hip popped back into the socket. I got on my bike and rode the rest of the way home. Later that night, however, I received a phone call and as I walked toward the stairs where I would answer the telephone, I collapsed. My hip dislocated for good. Shortly thereafter, I was told that because of the spina bifida, I didn't have enough muscle to hold my hip in its socket and I would need to undergo surgery.

Over the next 12 months, I endured five major hip operations and spent my time lying in a body cast. We sold our piano so that we could fit a hospital bed in the living room and this was where I stayed when I wasn't in the hospital. We didn't have a remote control for our TV, so I was usually at the mercy of my sister or three brothers when it came to watching TV. The telephone wasn't always accessible, either, although I didn't have the privacy I would have liked anyway because I was in the main room of the house.

One of the hardest things to think about was the amount of school I was missing. I had a tutor; however, she couldn't teach me the algebra and geometry I needed to know because she didn't know it herself. She gave me assignments in U.S. and world history as well as English, but it just wasn't the same as being in school. I didn't want to repeat the year I was missing in school because I wanted to be with my friends when I returned.

On the positive side of things, I did make some great friends while in the hospital. They were primarily the nurses who took care of me at Milwaukee Children's Hospital. When I wasn't in the hospital, I would call the nurses that gave me their home phone numbers at least once a week and make plans for my next hospital visit. The telephone became my "lifeline" to the outside world.

After I had my final body cast removed, I was sent home and told to work on gaining some flexibility back in my hips and knees. I was also supposed to work on sitting up in bed. This was easier said than done after spending all that time in a body cast. After about three weeks, I went back to the hospital to have some x-rays taken and to see my doctor. Little did I know I was about to receive news that would take many years to accept. My hip was dislocating again. After all the surgeries, the fact still remained that I didn't have enough muscle in my lower body to hold my hip in its socket. I was devastated, angry, resentful, and very depressed. Why had I lost an entire year of my life for no reason? I was now going to have to walk not only with braces, but with crutches, too. Even worse than that, I was going to have to get my first wheelchair so that I could cover longer distances independently.

I returned to school six weeks after realizing I was now going to need crutches and a wheelchair. I wasn't accepting the idea of a wheelchair yet and I didn't have the ability to make others feel comfortable with it either. When I returned to school, many of the students didn't know how to act around me. Now, Jean was using a wheelchair. Their reactions made me sad. My confidence in the classroom also plummeted. When I sat in on my first geometry class, I was completely lost. I was lucky to pass the class with a "D." English had always been a favorite subject of mine; however, while sitting and listening to the instructor, I wondered what language he was speaking. He was talking about iambic pentameters and tetrameters (meter used in poetry). I thought about asking, "Excuse me, could you start over?" Needless to say, I barely made it out of that semester and decided to switch schools for my junior and senior years.

While at the new high school, I met another kid who had been born with spina bifida and used a wheelchair. He is the person who introduced me to wheelchair sports. He asked me if I had ever heard of wheelchair soccer. My reaction was "Wheelchair soccer? How do you play that? You need your legs to play soccer!" He proceeded to tell me it was an adapted game and he was part of a team that practiced on Saturdays. When I heard the word "adapted," warning signals went up all over the place. I figured it was probably something hokey and non-competitive. Besides, I didn't want to hang out with those "wheelchair people." I wasn't one of them and I wasn't about to become one of them either. After a year of being nagged and prodded, I finally decided I would go to one practice. I knew I wouldn't like it, but at least it would get this kid off my back. I was quite surprised when I started practicing and playing with the other people there. Wheelchair soccer wasn't hokey at all! It was very competitive! I liked it! People were incredibly aggressive and some of the kids were getting knocked out of their chairs. The staff working the practice didn't get frantic or panicked when bodies were flying around because they knew that was the nature of sport. What a liberating activity! After all the years of watching my sister bring home basketball trophies, I was going to have the opportunity to "get in there and get dirty too!" My parents were not as excited with the idea as I was, particularly when I started coming home with parts broken off my wheelchair. Fortunately, the staff of the soccer program talked my parents into allowing me to continue participating. With the help of insurance money, I got rid of my hospital chair and bought a sports chair.

After my experience with wheelchair soccer, the whole world of athletics seemed to open up to me. I became involved in wheelchair football, softball, tennis, racquetball, ice hockey, basketball, etc. You name the sport, it could be done. I discovered water skiing and even learned how to square dance!

During this time of athletic awakening, I had graduated from high school and begun college. I didn't realize it at the time, but I was using sport as a way to escape the things that were bothering me, much like people become lost in their work or alcohol. Although sport was a great thing, I still wasn't dealing with my disability very well. I still saw it as a bad and limiting thing. I hated the disability and I hated myself. At the same time, my parents were going through a divorce and that situation took its toll on me as well. After three semesters of college work, I flunked out of school. The only thing I had been able to control throughout my life was now another thing that was out of my control. I did not want to be alive.

Fortunately, one of the nurses I met while in the hospital became a godsend. She invited me to come live with her for a year as a nanny and to help take care of her 14-month-old son and 2-1/2-year-old daughter. She was going back to school and her husband had been working 14-hour days to help make financial ends meet. I jumped at the offer. It was then that I learned how busy day-to-day childcare can be (not that I didn't have fun)!

I still was able to stay involved in wheelchair sports during my year of "nanny-hood" because most of the activities were held at night and the majority of my responsibilities with the children took place during the day. About three months into my new living arrangement, I attended a wheelchair sports workshop held in Milwaukee. One of the speakers invited to participate was Dr. Brad Hedrick. He was the supervisor of the Recreation and Athletics Program for Students with Disabilities at the University of Illinois. He saw me playing an exhibition game of wheelchair soccer and came up to me afterward to see if I would be interested in attending the University of Illinois. He expressed an interest in having me be part of his women's wheelchair basketball team. Although I didn't think I was interested I gave him my phone number and address.

Over the next six months, Brad called and sent me letters. It was quite flattering to be so heavily recruited. The flattery I felt is probably why I started to think about his offer seriously. I knew I needed a change in my life and I wasn't sure of what I was going to do after my year of working as a nanny had ended. The more I thought about going to school away from home, the more attractive it sounded. Six months after Brad made his offer, I applied to school. I didn't get accepted right away. I was told I had to go back to school for a semester to prove that I could handle a college course load. So, that is what I did in the spring of 1987, and by the fall I had moved to Champaign, Illinois, to begin my collegiate sports career.

Sports, Everyone!

Although the University of Illinois has some athletic scholarship money currently for students with disabilities, it was not available when I arrived on campus. I had to borrow money from my grandmother to help cover the cost of out-of-state tuition until I could apply for residency (and be accepted) in the state of Illinois. My move to Illinois was tough financially, athletically, and socially. I not only participated in basketball but also in track and road racing. I had been to track nationals during the summer of 1987 and won five gold medals on two months of training. Because of my success at nationals, I was invited to be a part of the U.S. Developmental Track Team competing in England one month later. My sponsor, the Derse Company, paid the $2000 fee for me to travel overseas for this competition. I ended up winning nine gold medals.

I had met the University of Illinois track coach, Marty Morse, during the summer of 1987 and knew I would probably be training under him as well as under Brad Hedrick. Between the weight training three times a week, the basketball practices six to seven days a week, and the track and road racing six to seven days a week, I had barely enough time left for schoolwork. I learned time management in a hurry! There was no way I would allow myself to flunk out of school again and there was no way I would allow myself to miss any workouts. This situation left me with no time to socialize or get to know people outside of class. It was a rough transition for me and I wondered if I hadn't made a bad decision in moving to Illinois.

It took me two years before I could say I actually liked it in Illinois. My success did not come easily once I arrived on campus. I was no longer surrounded by developmental or recreational athletes. I was among some of the most elite athletes in the world. For example, Sharon Hedrick had won an Olympic gold medal in the 1984 Los Angeles Olympic Games. Ann Cody held national records in the 5000m and 10,000m events on the track. Both women had played wheelchair basketball at the national level and they were good! Additionally, after moving to Champaign, I realized that Marty Morse was the top racing coach in the nation and among the best in the world. I learned humility quickly.

In 1988, I had dreams of making the Olympic team that was traveling to Seoul, South Korea. Beginning with the 1984 Los Angeles Olympics, two Olympic Exhibition Events have been held for wheelchair athletes: an 800m event for women and a 1500m event for men. Although I had been only training seriously for nine months, I believed I would make the Olympic team based on my performances the previous year. I was wrong. I ended up being the second alternate, which meant two people would have to decide against going to the Olympics in order for me to attend. I felt frustrated. I looked back over the nine months I had been in Illinois and thought I had sacrificed too many things to not be going to Korea. I had to make a decision as to whether I was going to give myself a realistic chance to develop and realize my potential or return to Milwaukee and find something else to do. I decided to give myself another four years to prepare for the 1992 Olympic Games that would be held in Barcelona, Spain. Besides, I did have two teammates from Illinois (Ann and Sharon) who would be representing the U.S.A. in Korea and they had done a lot more work over the five years than I had done. I watched their race on TV a few months later and saw Sharon win her second gold medal. Ann finished fifth in a very tight race for the bronze medal.

My first two years on the University of Illinois Women's Wheelchair Basketball Team were very successful, despite the fact there were four of us freshmen who arrived on campus at the same time. We were runners-up in the national championship games both years, losing to a team from Minnesota in 1988 and 1989.

When not on the basketball court with Brad (or in class), I was in the wright room, on the track, on the road, or on the rollers with Marty. (Rollers are cylinders that allow wheelchair athletes to push in place, indoors, when the weather is not conducive to pushing outside.) Marty had been trying to talk me into doing a marathon during my first two years on campus but I thought his suggestion was a little crazy. I arrived at the university as a sprinter. I felt that an 800m (or 1/2-mile) event was the longest distance I wanted to go on the track and a 10K (or 6.2 miles) was the longest I wanted to go on the road. After I won my first national level roadrace (a 7.4-mile event), my mind started to change.

My first marathon was the 1989 Chicago Marathon. Basketball practices had resumed and I was feeling exhausted. About the time I finished the work required for the marathon it would be time to go to basketball practice. In my mind, this was going to be the only marathon I would ever do. I ended up finishing in second place, about one minute behind Ann Cody. I was satisfied with that. However, Marty came up to me as excited as ever, saying "Do you realize what you've just done?! You've qualified for the Boston Marathon!" My reaction was not one of excitement. I really didn't want to do it. I didn't want to do the work and I didn't want to do the race. Sometimes, however, when a coach strongly suggests something, the athlete ends up going along with the suggestion. Therefore, while preparing for the National Women's Wheelchair Basketball Championships, I was also preparing for the Boston Marathon which would be held less than two weeks later. (Ann Cody attempted the same feat.)

Our basketball team won the 1990 National Championships. We enjoyed the victory tremendously. In between our games on the basketball court, though, Ann and I would jump into our racing chairs and do a workout on the rollers that were set up in our hotel room. We were in great shape! Actually, I thought Ann was in better shape than I. When we returned to Champaign briefly before flying out to Boston, I could not keep up with her during our workouts. If we would do a 20-mile push, she would finish several minutes ahead of me. For this reason alone, I did not feel I belonged in the Boston Marathon. Even while we sat on the start line, I questioned why I was there. I didn't think I was strong enough to do this race and I didn't want to embarrass myself. Most of all, I didn't want any woman who had never before beaten me to get the best of me on the Boston course.

The gun went off and, whether I liked it or not, I was competing in my first Boston Marathon. I was happy to have jumped in with the lead pack of women. In wheelchair racing, we utilize a tactic called drafting. Cyclists use it, car racers use it and wheelchair racers use it. Basically, it's a form of tailgating. A line forms behind the person who is in front of everyone else. The person in front is breaking the wind for others behind him or her and thus, the athletes "in the draft" don't have to work as hard while they're pushing. They get "pulled along" by the person in front and are conserving their energy. (In wheelchair racing, it is illegal for men and women to draft each other as it is illegal for paraplegics and quadriplegics to draft one another.)

Theoretically, everyone in the drafting pack is supposed to take a turn pulling up front. However, that doesn't always happen and it sometimes can cause some discord between the athletes. Fortunately, the drafting pack that had formed was one in which each of three women were taking their turn at the head of the pack. The pack consisted of Ann Cody, Connie Hansen (an athlete from Denmark), and me. At the nine-mile mark, Ann made a break away from Connie and me. After that, I chose to slow the pace down because I wanted Ann to lengthen her lead; we wanted an "Illinois person" to win the race. Every time Connie went up to the front she would pull as hard as she could. However, when I went to the front, I dropped the speed about 1 m.p.h. Ann disappeared ahead of us.

When Connie and I arrived at the 17 mile mark near Wellesley College, we took a right turn and began climbing the steepest hill on the Boston course (the infamous Heartbreak Hill is the longest). Much to my surprise, I had created a gap between Connie and me. When I got to the top of the hill, I looked behind me and noticed Connie was about 50 meters behind me. I had an immediate adrenaline rush. The next three miles I pushed as hard as I could because I didn't want Connie to catch me. During this time, I noticed I was getting closer to Ann. I caught her at the bottom of Heartbreak Hill (around mile 20). She had me go up to the front and pull since it appeared I had a little more energy. After about two minutes, I started getting tired and turned around to ask her to move up to the front. It was then that I realized I had already out-climbed her by about 25 meters and I should keep on going. I couldn't believe it! I was actually winning this race! And to think I didn't even believe I belonged in it! I went on to win the race and set a new world record of 1 hour, 43 minutes, 17 seconds. It was an incredible ending to an incredible race; I broke the world record by six minutes!

The rest of my racing season wasn't as dramatic as my race in Boston; however, 1990 was the start of bigger things to come. In the fall, I began my final season of basketball. With one national championship under our belts, the University of Illinois was hungry for another one. As the spring of 1991 rolled around, my schedule became as hectic as it had been the previous year. Not only did I have to help defend our national basketball title, but I also had to defend my Boston Marathon win. Just as Ann and I had trained in between the ballgames in 1990, so we also trained in between the ballgames in 1991. The only difference was we were in Southern California and thus able to do our 20 mile pushes along the beach. Similar to the year before, Ann was again having stronger workouts than I. We won our second consecutive basketball championship with at least as much excitement and emotion as the first championship victory. The Boston Marathon was in less than two weeks, though, so our euphoria didn't last long.

As I sat on the start line in the 1991 Boston event, I reflected on the training I had done to prepare for this event. I was unsure if it was possible to repeat as the winner. I had wanted my training to be stronger. Actually, I wanted a couple more weeks to get ready. But as the gun went off, I automatically started my second Boston Marathon.

This year's race was completely different from last year's event. Connie, Ann, and I worked together again but we all stayed together until the hill at mile 17. At that point I broke away and knew I just had to keep pushing hard. I didn't know what was happening between Ann and Connie; I was hoping Ann was having a strong day. I went on to win my second Boston Marathon with my second consecutive world record. The feeling as I crossed the finish line was still one of euphoria. Winning doesn't get old when you work hard.

The excitement didn't end at Boston that year. I successfully finished my first semester of graduate work in Rehabilitation Administration after having graduated with a bachelor's degree (with honors) in Speech Communication. I took a lot of pride in the academic accomplishments because the ghost of flunking out of school never left my mind. It felt good to have regained control of my academic career.

Athletically, I went on to break national and world records later that summer in the 800m and 1500m events on the track and in the 10K event on the road. What a year! I was really beginning to like racing!

Some time in July of that year I received a call from the Women's

Sports Foundation. I wasn't familiar with who they were but I was informed that I had been nominated for their Sudafed Amateur Sportswoman of the Year Award. Little did I know this was an organization that had been formed by great athletes like Billie Jean King (the tennis legend) and Donna DeVarona (the accomplished Olympic swimmer). It was a larger honor to have been nominated than I realized. Athletes who have received this award include Jackie Joyner-Kersee, Tracy Austin, Janet Evans, and Bonnie Blair.

One month later, they called me back to tell me I had made the list for the top ten athletes who were still in the running for this award. I asked them who the other athletes on the list were and I was given names like Karen and Sarah Josephson (Olympic synchronized swimmers), Donna Weinbrecht (Olympic mogul skier), Kristi Yamaguchi (Olympic figure skater), and the list went on. I remember thinking that it was an honor to have made the "top ten list"; however, I thought there was no way I would ever win this prestigious award. I was wrong. One month after I was told I had been one of the ten finalists, I was told I had been chosen for the award. It gave me goose bumps when I received the call. I couldn't believe I had actually been chosen to receive the award!

The awards banquet was held in October in New York City. It was a black tie event that had attracted the attention of the NBC show "Entertainment Tonight." I had never been in attendance at a black tie affair before and felt nervous about my first experience. I was seated at a table that had been bought out by ESPN so I had the opportunity to meet several fun personalities. Later that evening, Jackie Joyner-Kersee presented my award to me. I was handed the microphone and invited to make a few comments. I didn't speak long, but I do remember explaining how sport for the disabled has followed the same evolution as sport for women. People didn't accept it when it was first introduced. The general public didn't believe women could be so athletic, strong, or coordinated enough to participate in sport. It was thought, "They might get hurt." The media hasn't always been a strong supporter of women's sports either. Those same attitudes have followed athletes with disabilities.

I am thrilled the Women's Sports Foundation did not have the same biases as the general public. The award I received from them allowed me to know that I was recognized and respected as a legitimate elite athlete. I was not viewed as courageous; I was viewed as athletic. They realized the sacrifices I made to participate in sport at the level I did were not out of courage, but out of competitiveness and a desire to be the very best.

I think the greatest lesson I have learned during my tenure at the University of Illinois is that disability is a characteristic like height or skin color. One cannot choose how tall they become; they're forced to work with what they've got. Similarly, one cannot choose their skin color and therefore must learn their limits on how long they can be in the sun.

Disability is not a defining principle. Except in a small percentage of cases, it does not preclude people from having the normal life experiences of going to school, finding employment, participating in sport, getting married, etc. One can have a disability and not be disabled. Webster's Dictionary defines the word disabled as "incapacitated" or "powerless." That definition does not fit my lifestyle or the lifestyle of most of the 43 million Americans mentioned in the 1990 Americans with Disabilities Act. It is more a stigma than a definition.

My experience at the Women's Sports Foundation Banquet will forever be one of the highlights of my life. I didn't win the award because I had a disability. I won the award because I was an athlete who had achieved a high level in sport (such as back-to-back world records in the famed Boston Marathon).

As the calendar year turned to 1992, I knew I was in store for a busy year. The Boston Marathon was coming up again, but also the Olympic trials. I didn't have to worry about basketball anymore so my focus was entirely on training for Boston and the road races that came before it. Actually, I did have one occasion to deviate from my race preparation. I was asked to sing the National Anthem before the Milwaukee Brewers' Home Opener in April 1992. They were honoring Wisconsin Olympians at this game and invited me to sing the anthem since they knew I was preparing for the Summer Olympic Trials. I was quite nervous to be sure. I had never sung in front of 53,000 people before. In fact, I had only sung the anthem in public once before when the cities of Champaign and Urbana, Illinois, declared a "Jean Driscoll Day." (I sang the anthem before a women's basketball game at which I was honored in February of 1992.) It was a great experience, though. It wasn't a disability thing; it was a life experience thing.

A few weeks later, I returned to Boston and defended my title for the third consecutive year with my third consecutive world record. I am often asked if winning the Boston Marathon is becoming old and mundane; I always respond by asking if they think Bonnie Blair ever gets tired of accepting her Olympic gold medals. When you have to work hard to achieve a goal, the success doesn't get old!

My next goal was to qualify for the Olympic games and eventually, win the gold medal. The Olympic trials were in New Orleans and there were several races that had to be run before the final eight women and eight men would earn their positions in the Olympic Exhibition Events. My peak (or best performance condition) was timed perfectly and I ended up being the number one qualifier for the Olympic Event that would be held on August 2, 1992. Now I would have to return to Champaign and use the final three to four weeks before leaving for Europe to sharpen my fitness level and get mentally prepared to run a smart race.

The road to Barcelona began in Tampa, Florida, on July 20th. We went through a regimen called "processing" which meant we picked up our U.S. Olympic Issue (i.e. uniforms, shoes, dress sweats, Cabbage Patch dolls) and then went through a briefing on what to expect upon our arrival in Spain. Next we boarded a chartered flight which took us to Barcelona. When the plane landed, four other American wheelchair athletes and I were bused to France where we would train for a week and get used to the time change. The week went quickly and before we knew it, the time had come to travel back down to Barcelona.

The women's 800m event was run at 11:30 a.m. and the men's 1500m event was at 11:35 a.m. I had gone over the details of my race so many times in my head that I knew exactly what I had to do and where I had to make my move. Of course, during the course of my imagery, I won the gold medal and set the world record at least a million times!

The gun went off and I had a great start. In an 800m race, athletes have to stay in their assigned lanes until they reach a "break line" located 120 meters from the start line. At that point, if the track is clear, the athlete can move down into lane one enabling him or her to cover a smaller amount of distance around the track than one who is in an outside lane. I was the first one to the break line and quickly moved down into lane one. Connie Hansen, my rival from Denmark, jumped in my draft shortly thereafter. A second pack of women had formed on the outside of us so I knew Connie was trapped behind me. I didn't mind doing all the pulling because I knew Connie would have a difficult time getting out of her position. With about 210 meters to go, however, Connie somehow got out of the trap she was in and came flying around me. I was shocked for an instant and then started working to close the one second she had on me. When I realized the race was almost over and I wouldn't be able to close the gap on Connie, I let up on my final sprint a little. Suddenly, an athlete from Sweden swung out of my draft and nearly stole the silver medal from me. I ended up edging her out by 1/100 of a second. Never again will I let up in a final sprint!

I was disappointed at not meeting my goal of winning the gold medal and setting the world record. (Connie achieved both of those honors.) I did, however, set a new American record. My mother and aunt were there to see my first Olympic race. I received my Olympic silver medal from the queen of Spain. Again, it wasn't a disability thing; it was an Olympic thing.

One month later, I returned to Barcelona to compete in the Paralympics. The Paralympics are Olympic style competition for all athletes with disabilities. Athletes with varying disabilities compete against other athletes with similar disabilities (i.e., athletes who use wheelchairs compete against athletes who use wheelchairs, visually impaired runners compete against visually impaired runners, etc.). The sports contested in the Paralympic Games parallel the sports contested in the Olympic Games. In most cases the same sites and venues are used for both events and people from all over the world compete to earn the title of "best in the world."

I did not do well in the 1992 Paralympic Games. I was "burned out" from the emotion of the Boston Marathon, the Olympic Trials, and the Olympic event itself. I didn't make the finals in any of my races including the 800m event. I didn't come away with any world or national titles; that was hard to accept. I survived the event, though, and sometimes that can be the biggest goal.

Since 1992, I have been blessed with two more victories and two more world records in the Boston Marathon. Each race has its own drama and every victory is sweet and euphoric. Winning has not gotten old. Conversely, winning has given me the opportunity to do many things I might not have otherwise had the opportunity to do. I am mostly referring to speaking. I have been given an incredible platform on which to address the general public about life and disability. I get to share with them that disability is not a lifelong tragedy (although attitude can be). By talking about the many things I have done, it is harder to find things I haven't done. I have shared the speaking platform with Tom Landry and Isiah Thomas. I have gone jogging with President Clinton (all winners of the Boston Marathon are invited to run with him). I have a disability, but I haven't been incapacitated by it. When I am asked to sign autographs, I usually write, "Dream Big and Work Hard!" It's a tenet by which most everyone on this earth can live.

You Can Get Involved!

by Kirk M. Bauer

Kirk Bauer is Executive Director of Disabled Sports USA.

Whether you are disabled or a volunteer or professional who wants to help out, there are plenty of opportunities for you to become involved. As *Sports, Everyone!* shows, even those with a severe disability can participate in a wide range of activities, with the right equipment and trained instructors. The number and type of activities offered vary widely among communities, but they are growing everywhere and with a little initiative, you too can lead an active lifestyle!

The recently passed Americans With Disabilities Act (ADA) and the Individuals With Disabilities Education Act (IDEA) will provide the impetus for expanding recreation programs across the country. Under the ADA and IDEA, more and more schools, ski areas, fitness clubs, community recreation programs, boating facilities, and others will have to make "reasonable accommodations" for those with disabilities.

As a *recreationalist* with a disability, you can become involved through participation with local community sports organizations, such as the chapters of Disabled Sports USA (DS/USA). You can also participate in recreation programs run by local and regional municipalities, or through the schools. Swimming is still the most popular activity available, but many municipalities are starting to accommodate individuals in the full range of recreational activities.

If *competition* is your goal, become involved with one of the recognized Disabled Sports Organizations of the US Olympic Committee, such as DS/USA, or one of the other sports groups offering regional, national, and international competition opportunities. Through the USOC recognized organizations, athletes can establish their own training accounts and receive tax deductible contributions to help them defer the cost of training.

Everyone, disabled or not, can become involved as volunteers and professional instructors. Opportunities abound to volunteer with local community-based programs, that are either sports specific or are part of a larger nondisabled sports and recreation program. All the activities listed in this book are conducted by one of these organizations and they need your help! For more information, contact the local DS/USA chapter in your area or chapters of other sports organizations.

Funding is always a challenge when you are a volunteer or staff working to build a national or community-based organization, or an individual athlete seeking support for you training efforts. There never seem to be enough resources, financial or otherwise, to meet the needs, but there is help!

Many groups depend upon support from individuals through memberships and donations. Special events which help raise money, such as fun runs, auctions, ski races, and hole-in-one tournaments, can be planned and conducted. Civic organizations, such as Kiwanis, Shriners, and Lions Clubs, often help support organizations providing services for disabled individuals. Veterans' organizations, such as Paralyzed Veterans of America and Disabled American veterans, are also supportive of groups providing services to disabled veterans and others.

More and more, corporations are starting to support sports events, both because it helps the community and provides highly visible recognition of the corporate sponsor.

If you are involved in fund-raising, be sure to plan *at least* six months to one year ahead. Have a clear game plan and comprehensive budget. Learn about the funding sources you are approaching and seek out those whose guidelines fit your activities and objectives. Try to secure a personal, face-to-face meeting with your potential source, followed by simple, well written proposals. Personal meetings always produce the best results.

Also, be sure to register your group with the appropriate state charity bureau or similar agency. This is necessary if you are fund-raising for a public charity.

If you are involved with a community sports group, look for ways to **share resources** with other community groups and your local municipal recreation program. The future of sports and recreation for disabled individuals will depend greatly on partnerships which more efficiently utilize **existing resources** in the community.

The mission of Disabled Sports USA is clear: To help ensure physically disabled people of all ages have access to sports, recreation and physical education programs, from primary school through college, to the elite sports level and at the community level. Groups like DS/USA can help this process by developing adapted teaching techniques, developing adapted equipment and by working as partners with others to conduct programs.

More and more, this responsibility will and should be assumed by the community recreation programs, school physical education and sports programs and National Governing Bodies of the U.S. Olympic Committee; but we all have the responsibility to help this process.

Paralyzed Veterans of America

by Jim Angelo, Publications Manager, PVA

The Paralyzed Veterans of America (PVA) was founded following World War II with the vision of a better life for paralyzed veterans and others who face the daily challenge of life with a disability. At the outset, PVA founders were concerned about a wide range of issues—from improving Veterans Administration hospital conditions for spinal cord injury patients to developing meaningful therapy programs and other rehabilitation services.

At the same time, many PVA members wanted to continue their involvement in the sports and athletic competition they enjoyed prior to their injury. For many this took the form of wheelchair basketball, the first formally organized wheelchair sport.

PVA members and other veterans with disabilities were the active participants and driving forces behind the formation of many of the first wheelchair basketball teams. Following close behind came wheelchair track and field, and a host of other wheelchair sports. These sporting events were and still are sponsored by PVA and its chapters. National sports programs are funded through money authorized by PVA's Board of Directors and, in many cases, supplemented by corporate sponsorship.

The goal of these activities is to provide a means of improving the health, independence and self-image of paralyzed veterans and other people with disabilities through promoting and increasing their participation in sports, recreation, and fitness activities. From the initial strengthening of little-used muscle groups to developing wheelchair mobility skills, PVA believes that meaningful participation in wheelchair sports is one of the best tools for rehabilitation—both physical and emotional. Active participation in sports and recreation activities also creates a positive image and role models for others with disabilities.

Because of its value in rehabilitation, PVA actively encourages its members and others with disabilities to participate in the many sports and recreation activities it sponsors. Events range from local and regional to national. PVA helps each person rise to the highest level he or she wishes. Some ultimately choose sports as a career. And some reach the highest levels in international competition. One example is PVA member Kater Cornwell.

Cornwell, a paraplegic, was shot in Vietnam and later developed a viral infection that resulted in paralysis. Participating in sports was a big part of his rehabilitation. Cornwell has become a world-class athlete in weightlifting. He has been the USA National Champion five times in Division I of the heavyweight class. He also won gold medals at three World Championships and finished fifth in weightlifting in the Barcelona Paralympics. Since 1983, he has participated in the National Veterans Wheelchair Games—the largest such annual event in the country. Cornwell is a wonderful role model for both the able-bodied and people with disabilities. His "battle cry" declared before every weightlifting competition, "I will not be defeated," truly exemplifies his attitude to life.

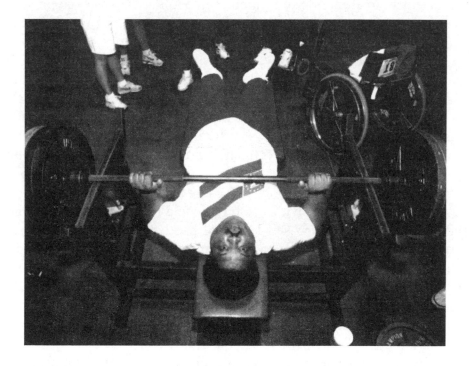

Kater Cornwell competing at the National Veterans Wheelchair Games

Today, in an effort to provide sports and recreational opportunities to meet the diverse needs of its members, PVA, through its Sports and Recreation Program, is a sponsor of every major national wheelchair sports championship in the United States. And PVA lobbies appropriate federal agencies and national sports and recreation organizations to incorporate equal programming for, and services to, people with disabilities, including the elimination of barriers to participation in existing programs.

PVA also supports such organizations as Wheelchair Sports USA (formerly NWAA), the National Wheelchair Basketball Association (NWBA), the National Foundation for Wheelchair Tennis (NFWT), the American Wheelchair Bowling Association (AWBA) and the 1996 Paralympics, which will be held in Atlanta, Georgia. In addition, PVA has been a leader in supporting the growth of emerging sports such as quad rugby, which now is the fastest growing team sport for quadriplegics.

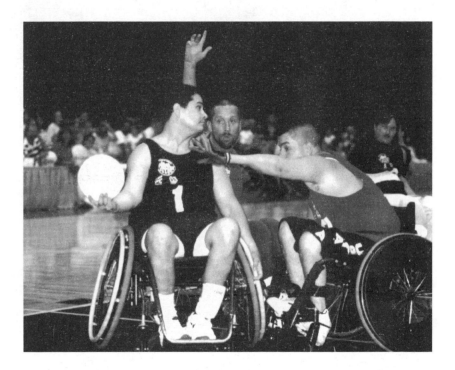

PVA-sponsored Quad Rugby Tournament

Through its Sports and Recreation Program, PVA also provides opportunities for novice athletes and coaches to develop their skills and enhance their appreciation of selected sports in noncompetitive, educational programs such as the NWBA/PVA National Basketball Camp, NFWT/PVA National Tennis Training Camp, National Handicapped Sports Learn-to-Ski Clinics and PVA Quad Rugby Clinics.

PVA also sponsors and produces educational materials designed to provide coaches, athletes and others interested in wheelchair sports with the latest information on sports, equipment and training. In addition, PVA publishes *Sports 'n Spokes*, a full-color magazine that covers the exciting and colorful events and personalities of wheelchair sports.

For almost 50 years, sports and recreation have played an integral part in PVA. PVA believes that sports and recreation provide its members and others with disabilities an important element in rehabilitation, as well as the opportunity to live life to the fullest.

PVA National Bass Trail: This year the trail expanded to five tournaments. This angler with disabilities shows his catch at the Potomac Classic, part of the PVA National Bass Trail.

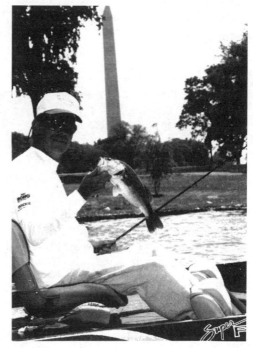

Profile: Shad Dahlgren

By Shad Dahlgren

Shad Dahlgren is a student athlete at the University of Nebraska who pioneered wheelchair basketball.

The following is my perception of disabled athletics. To truly understand that perception, a person must understand where I came from and how I was raised, so that is where I started.

I grew up on a farm near the small community of Bertrand, Nebraska. Being raised on a farm is ridiculed by many people but I say it with pride. On the farm I learned what many kids today don't: a good work ethic and responsibilities of the day-to-day care of animals. The attitude and the ethics that I learned on the farm have allowed me to overcome my disability and get back on the road to success.

As a little kid I rode the tractor with my dad, harvesting corn every Saturday in the fall. On Saturdays in the fall all farmers harvesting, and all of Nebraska, are tuned into Lincoln's Memorial Stadium as the Cornhuskers do battle on the football field. On that tractor, looking up at my dad, I learned learn to anticipate those immortal words of "touchdown, touchdown, touchdown," beaming from the radio. From this early age, I learned the importance of athletics to my dad and many other people in small towns. For athletics are the only real chance small towns have of being a place people remember instead of just another dot on a map.

In my first two years of high school I was an average athlete, not great but not terrible. However, I liked athletics and loved the spirit of competition. I was looking forward to my last two years of high school athletics, but all that changed on a warm summer evening in June. On June 3, 1990, I rolled my car on a gravel road, I was thrown out and dislocated a vertebrae in my back. The accident was caused by my own carelessness and disrespect for the gravel roads I grew up on. I was flown to Immanuel Hospital in Omaha where I spent the entire summer adjusting to life in a wheelchair.

Upon my return home I began my junior year of high school just as if there was no summer break at all, only now I was seated in a wheelchair. As a senior I watched my former teammates win two state championships. People I once played alongside of were now heroes of the town. They had put Bertrand on the map and all I could do was painfully watch.

In the summer of 1992 I moved to Lincoln and enrolled in Southeast Community College, majoring in computers. As luck would have it, the first day I moved to town I ran into the wife of a man who was in a wheelchair and heavily involved in disabled athletics. I contacted him and he got me involved with a group that played wheelchair basketball, known as Handicapped Recreational Service. I played basketball one time and I was hooked. I had been starved of athletics for two years, never knowing that disabled athletics existed, and now I had found them. I went crazy playing all the time and venting two years of frustration built up by watching athletics instead of playing.

In January of 1993 I became a student at the University of Nebraska majoring in General Agriculture. Shortly after that I was recruited by Lew Shaver of Southwest State University in Marshall, Minnesota, to play wheelchair basketball for him. This was a major turning point in my life and attitude towards life in a wheelchair. Someone now wanted me for my physical skills and ability. This was a turning point because it was not an offer made out of pity or charity, but out of a legitimate need. Because of this the offer was very tempting; however I loved the University of Nebraska and what I was studying so I decided to not play for SSU. With the decision I knew that I had turned down a great opportunity, one of playing athletics on the college level. So with the thought of this great school with the great athletic tradition I started the first disabled athletic team at the University of Nebraska in the fall of 1993.

The team is now competing on the national level and is gaining considerable recognition from the community and state. The team members consider themselves as role models for the disabled youth of Nebraska. This is the team's most rewarding aspect because it gives the youth something to strive for. They can now feel the enthusiasm of athletics that other kids do in hopes that they someday will play for the University of Nebraska and become a Husker. In addition it keeps them from the depression that can result from their disability, depression that may lead to drug abuse as too many disabled are led.

My personal purpose in disabled athletics is to show the people who play and the people who spectate that athletics and the world are 99% mental. This is nowhere more evident than in disabled athletics, where a group of people are using 50% of their body to accomplish a common goal—the same goal that all other people use in regular athletics. The mind is the common factor of both. If more people become aware of this then disabilities will be looked upon differently, they will be looked upon as totally equal as they should be.

Profile: Jim Mastro

by Jennifer Hester

Jim Mastro is a world class athlete and Ph.D. who is also blind.

It's difficult to talk about Jim Mastro without mentioning sports. The 46-year-old has been competing for most of his life in one sport or another—despite the fact that he's totally blind. "I guess it's the love of sports that motivates Jim," says Cheryl Mastro, Jim's wife of more than 20 years. "He's always enjoyed sports as long as I've known him, and he enjoys working with other people." That love for sports took him a long way: to the 1976 Olympic team as an alternate, the first World University Games, 15 world championships, every Paralympic Games since 1976, nine Paralympic medals in four sports and collegiate championships.

It began with gymnastics, track and field and wrestling for the Minnesota native. Then blind in only one eye, he excelled in the athletic arena. His build, he said, was perfect for the sports: 180 pounds of muscle his junior year of high school.

But his days as a high school athlete were to come to a stop between his junior and senior years. Mastro, born blind in his right eye, lost the sight in his left eye from a detached retina, the result of an injury sustained when he was 11.

"When I went blind, I didn't really compete in anything for two years," he recalled. "I decided to go back out for wrestling when I got to college. It was driving me crazy, frankly, that I wasn't doing anything in competition or in sports."

He returned to wrestling, this time on the college level, at Augsburg College in Minnesota. He suffered his share of defeats in his return to the sport, but, like any good athlete, Mastro learned from the experiences. "I learned how hard I was going to have to go to do well," he said. "Anybody can just do it for fun, but if you want to do well, you have to know how far you have to go."

Mastro went as far as he could on the collegiate level: to the conference and national championships. In 1972, he won the conference at 177 lbs. "I decided that I wanted to continue wrestling, and I kept going with it," he said. "My senior year in college there were trials for the U.S. team to the World University Games—the first World University Games that they had. I won the national championship, and I was on the United States team."

Mastro went on to make the U.S. Olympic Greco-Roman wrestling team as an alternate in 1976. "Even though I had placed nationally a number of times, they didn't think a blind guy could beat up on all those sighted guys," he said. "That was one of my big accomplishments."

"It's not at all uncommon for people to be really surprised when a blind athlete is successful," said Charlie Huebner, executive director of the United States Association of Blind Athletes (USABA). "Part of what we do at USABA is try to change the stereotype that people like Jim can't compete and can't be successful just because they're blind. People who are blind can accomplish just as much as everyone else." Mastro says that stereotypes such as these encouraged him to return to sports in the first place. "One of the things that was interesting was that because I was blind, they didn't think I could compete," he said of his return to wrestling. "So I decided to try it anyway."

After so many accomplishments in wrestling, in his late 20s Mastro decided to move on to other sports. In the late 1970s and early '80s, he started with track and field and competed for the first time since high school in shotput, discus, and javelin. He also added goalball, an indoor team sport for blind athletes, to his activities.

In 1980, the all-around athlete made the U.S. team in wrestling, goalball, and track and field to compete at the International Games for the Disabled. He came home with a gold medal in wrestling and a silver in goalball. He broke world records three times earning his silver medal in shotput.

Mastro went on to add judo to his accomplishments when, in 1986, the USABA put on at the Braille Institute a demonstration in judo. "And I thought, 'I can do this. Judo is really Greco-Roman wrestling with your jammies on.'" Despite some technique differences, the moves in the two sports are extraordinarily similar, Mastro said. "There are some subtle differences, like chokes and arm bars and things like that. But wrestling for almost 20 years, I was doing some of the judo moves."

He was proven right. The recent notches on his third degree black belt include gold medals at the 1995 World Judo Championships, 1994 BAJA International Judo Tournament and 1992, 1993, and 1994 USABA National Championships. He also won silver medals at the 1992 Paralympics and the 1991 International Judo Championships.

Perhaps it is the discovery of such success, extraordinary for any athlete, that motivates Mastro now to involve blind children in sports. While it is becoming less rare for blind children to compete in the athletic arena, Mastro said he thinks attitudes still haven't changed enough from when he was a blind college athlete. "Coaches are still not going out there and looking for blind kids out in their hallway and saying, 'Hey, you should be on our wrestling team,' or 'Hey, you should be on our swim team.' It's up to the individuals to go out there and do it for themselves. They've got to want to go out there and do it."

"Blind athletes like Jim Mastro have discovered for themselves what it means to be successful in sports," said USABA's Huebner. "Jim wants to share that feeling with kids who might not consider that they have the potential and the ability to do well because they may have been told all their lives that they can't."

Mastro's efforts to have coaches and educators include blind kids in sports is part of the reason he made it to the top in another part of the sports arena: physical education. In 1985, the national champion earned his Ph.D. in physical education with an emphasis on adapted and developmental physical education. His degree from Texas Women's University took four years of hard work to complete and has led to an associate teaching position at the University of Minnesota.

Like his entry into sports, however, Mastro has found that not everyone in physical education can immediately accept a blind man in a field that seems to rely so heavily on the senses.

"I don't know if physical education people are ready for someone who is blind to be in physical education," he commented. "When you look at who makes up the committees and things like that, they're biochemists and all that kind of stuff who have a stereotype of what a blind person is. And that, for want of anything better, is a person selling pencils on a street corner, helpless, hopeless and that kind of thing.

"Well, in some areas, being visually impaired is not a big problem. But in the physical education area, I guess it is a problem. It's probably why I'm the only one."

While Mastro said his entry into the field has been difficult, it has also been rewarding. His position at the University of Minnesota allows him to hold sports camps for blind children.

"I suppose to see myself five or ten years from now would be me still trying to get more and more of the public to realize that kids who are blind or whatever should be involved with sports," he said. "And I imagine I'll be doing that forever."

25

Profile: Marcy Monasterial—The Oldest Olympian

Marcy Monasterial is a hall of fame table tennis competitor.

Marcy Monasterial is the nation's top-ranked table tennis player over the age of 70 in both able-bodied and disabled categories. Ranked #1 by the National Handicapped Sports in table tennis, Marcy is also ranked nationally by the United States Table Tennis Association (USTTA). Marcy was previously ranked #2 in the world in Class 10 (amputee below the elbow) and is the most dominant amputee table tennis player in the United States today. He is still a player to be reckoned with, even among able-bodied competitors.

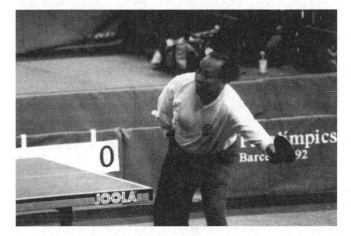

Marcy Monasterial at the 1992 Paralympic Games in Barcelona

Marcy has competed all over the world in no fewer than 22 counties. This includes the 1984 Paralympic Games in Uniondale, New York, where he won silver and bronze medals; the 1988 Paralympic games in Seoul, Korea, where he twice defeated the eventual men's singles gold medalist in round robin competition, and reached the quarter-finals; the 1987 Handicapped World Games in Paris, France, where he won a silver medal; and the 1992 Paralympic Games in Barcelona, Spain, where he won a bronze medal in Team Table Tennis.

Marcy's table tennis career and tournament competitions has spanned seven decades. In July 1993 in Laguna Hills, California, Marcy won the over-70 National Table Tennis Championships for both able-bodied and disabled. In 1994 he brought his tournament wins to more than 600. He was the U.S. Amputee Athletic Association Athlete of the Year in 1988-1989.

Marcy took undergraduate courses at Indiana University in 1945. He went on to Columbia University where he received a BS in Journalism and a dual Masters in Sociology and Library Science.

Marcy worked for 36 years at the United Nations as a Social Affairs Officer and Librarian before retiring in 1983. He then joined the editorial staff at a publishing company. This Sports Hall of Fame athlete is a father of four and grandfather of 3. He trains at the Burke Rehabilitation Center in White Plains, New York, with wheelchair table tennis athletes. He participated in the US Olympic Festival in July 1994 in St. Louis where he won a team gold medal in disabled table tennis. At 71, Marcy was the oldest ever at an Olympic Festival. With his exuberant personality and gripping personal story, Marcy was sought after by the press and other media at the Games.

"My age, how I got the disability, the fact that I'm diabetic—there were many things for them to touch upon. I was surrounded by so many notebooks and tape recorders for about an hour and a half. And each one (reporter) would come away with a different story," says Marcy.

Marcy grew up in the Philippines watching table tennis in a parlor across the street from his house. Using his right hand, he quickly found he had a knack for the game and went on to become a Philippine junior champion. When the Japanese invaded his country in World War II, Marcy and his brother went to work for the underground, delivering messages to the Americans. On one of these missions sentries ordered Marcy to halt and shot him as he ran away. At the hospital, his right arm was amputated.

Although Marcy can now joke about switching to his left arm because he didn't have a right hand anymore, in truth he faced depression at the time. But he fought on, teaching himself to play again with his left hand. Within three weeks he was playing again. But he never figured out how to realign his body and plays with a left backhand to replace his right forehand.

His prize possession is his paddle which he has had since 1944. It is the sole possession he has from his youth.

"I was the oldest at the 1984 Games. I was also the oldest at the 1988 Games in Seoul and in 1992 at Barcelona, and I'll be oldest one in Atlanta in 1996, God willing," says Marcy. He will be 73 then and has qualified for the Doubles Competition.

Sports Profile: Amputee Golf— A Sport for All Ages

First Swing

By Stephanie Martin

Reprinted by permission of The National Amputee Golf Association. This article originally appeared in the 1994 issue of Amputee Golfer Magazine.

The success of any endeavor can be measured in percentage gain. Consider then the success of the National Amputee Golf Association's "First Swing—Golf for the Physically Challenged" program: In 1988 three 2-day seminars were presented; in 1993 the number rose to 30, an increase of 1000%.

The First Swing program was developed to instruct therapists to teach and encourage the physically challenged to learn, or re-learn, the game of golf—not only because it is virtually the only sport every physically challenged individual, regardless of age, is able to play, but also because it contributes dramatically to the individual's emotional and physical well-being, instilling self-confidence and pride in personal achievement. It also enables the individual to enjoy the unique, friendly camaraderie found on the golf course. The program, thanks to the support by the PGA of America and the Disabled American Veterans Charitable Trust, has been offered free of cost to the hosting facility with respect to travel, room and board of the instructors.

Based on the premise that to play golf all one has to do is hit the ball, Bob Wilson, Executive Director of the Amputee Golf Association, a double below the knee amputee and devoted golfer, developed and perfected the program. The two-day seminar/clinic, hosted by rehabilitation hospitals, park and recreational departments of cities and towns, and prosthetic concerns, provides a learning forum for therapists and others interested in teaching the basics of the game to the Physically Challenged. The first day of the program is devoted to an instruction and learning course. The theory of golf and the singular differences presented by each physically challenged individual are discussed. Participants are invited to swing a club standing on one leg, sitting in a wheelchair, using only one hand, etc., to better appreciate the new demands that will be made on their educational training in teaching others. The second day is devoted to the therapists instructing the physically challenged participants under the tutelage of members of the National Amputee Golf Association's (NAGA) "First Swing" team.

The program is open to every physically challenged individual regardless of age or handicap. Children may begin by using a putter— excellent training for use in a game of miniature golf with friends. Adults may also take their first swing with a putter and then progress to a "Pitch and Putt" course or a Par-3 Executive layout. They may forego these intermediate steps, mastering the use of irons and woods in as short a time as possible in order to play on a local public or private course with friends and family.

Although not publicly advertised, word of this exceptional seminar does "get around," and either NAGA or Bob Wilson, personally, receive invitations from all over the country to present the program.

First Swing Goes International

Of singular note, the year also witnessed the inauguration of the First Swing going international. The Alberta Amputee Sports & Recreation Association requested that the First Swing be brought to Canada. Two seminars were held at Calgary and Toronto and were well attended by therapists and Canadian PGA golf professionals. The Canadian PGA also sanctioned the program for their professionals. It was interesting to note from comments made about the program, that golf is as popular in Canada as it is here in the States.

Program Recognized by the PGA of America . . .

In November 1992 NAGA received notification from the PGA of America Education Department that the "First Swing...Golf for the Physically Challenged" program had been approved for Continuing Education credit for PGA members who attend. This certification has been extended to 1994 seminars. NAGA hopes, what with the number of physically challenged in the U.S. pegged at 43 million, and the mandate of the Americans with Disabilities Act (ADA), that courses be accessible to the Physically Challenged, that PGA professionals will attend future seminars in order to become familiar with various disabilities and obtain the knowledge necessary to teach this segment of society. "Adopt a Hospital" is NAGA's battle cry and hopes that the PGA will echo the same within its ranks. "We are only in a particular area for two days," stated Bob Wilson, "who is better to take over and expand the program when we leave than a golf professional? From the hospital to the golf course is the goal."

In the past five years Bob Wilson and the NAGA instructional team have brought the program to over 2,500 therapists and physically challenged individuals. The number of people subsequently introduced or re-introduced by these trained therapists is unknown. But this we do know: The success of First Swing isn't measured solely in the percentage numbers indicated above. It is also measured in the number of lives touched. As the First Swing program expands its horizons throughout the United States and to other countries, the millions of physically challenged individuals who think they will never learn to play golf, or play golf again, will discover what they believe to be an impossibility can become a reality when they take their First Swing.

Sports Profile: Shooting Sports

NRA-Winchester Match Showcases Opportunities in Shooting Sports

by Dave Baskin, National Rifle Association

Printing by permission from Wheelchair Sports, USA

Disabled sport organizations are always searching for ways to promote their sports and thereby attract new athletes, for without a constant flow of new talent these groups will cease to exist. One way to interest potential athletes in disabled sports is to design introductory events which adequately challenge the participants and recognize the top performers for their efforts, while making sure to keep the competition fun. The National Rifle Association of America, through its NRA Disabled Shooting Services Department, has made a commitment to build interest and participation in the shooting sports for people with physical disabilities, on a grass roots level.

On March 10-13, 1994, the NRA conducted one of the most unique and important competition matches in its history at Camp ASCCA-Easter Seals, in Jackson's Gap, AL. The competition was held in conjunction with the Disabled Outdoor Organizations Recreation Symposium for over 200 representatives of disabled sportsmen groups and government fish and game agencies.

This match was designed in such a way as to provide both able-bodied competitors and those with physical disabilities an equal opportunity to fire their best score. All the competitors used the same rifle, which was loaned for the occasion by Lori Hoffman of Bensalem, PA. This particular gun was a .22 caliber German built Anschutz with a 12 power Leopold scope, and had been used by Lori to win the 1984 NRA Junior Smallbore Silhouette National Championship. The sensitivity of the light two-stage trigger on this rifle allowed shooters with hand dysfunction and finger problems the opportunity to compete. Many people who were unable to successfully operate a heavy standard type trigger were able to participate with the lighter, more sensitive trigger mechanism. This style trigger allowed several shooters to experience the independence of manually controlling the gun, instead of having to rely on a sip 'n puff device.

In order to further equalize the competition, all the shooters were required to fire the rifle from a special designed support stand which is used in international matches for the disabled. The stand is constructed with a spring just under the rifle-holding yoke, so that it only supports the weight of the gun and in no way enhances the stability factor. This design permitted each competitor to be challenged to the limit of their ability.

The NRA donated a set of their finest international grade medals and a carton of targets for this event. Winchester Division of the Olin Corporation gave a case of their high quality .22 rifle ammunition, which proved to be excellent and accounted for the many great scores that were fired in this match. At the conclusion of the competition, all the remaining targets and ammunition were donated by these two fine organizations to the Camp ASCCA-Easter Seals shooting program.

Twenty-nine people ventured out to the Camp ASCCA shooting range to test their skills in this NRA-Winchester Match.

Each competitor fired twenty record shots at the paper targets which were mounted thirty yards away. In order to score a maximum of ten points for each shot, the shooter had to hit the center ring of the target, which was the size of a nickel. The "X count" was used for breaking any scoring ties and was a small ring the size of a pencil eraser inside the ten ring. The best possible score that anyone could shoot would be a perfect 200 points with 20 "X's."

The match winning score of 200-17X was fired by Hope Kelly of Birmingham, AL. Hope demonstrated a lot of determination and patience, and as a result took home a beautiful NRA Gold Medal for her effort.

Don Basye from Temperance, MI, was the very last shooter to roll up to the firing line just as early evening shadows were closing in upon the range. In spite of the added problem of having to shoot the right-handed rifle from the left side, Don's powers of concentration carried him to a very fine silver medal winning score of 200-16X.

The competition for some of the following positions was so close that a tie-breaking system had to be brought into play. Whenever the points and "X count" was tied, we compared each competitor's last 5-shot string until the tie was broken. Such a process was used to determine third place for Jack East of Little Rock, AR, and fourth for John Kopchik from Chicago, IL, as both men shot identical scores of 200-15X.

Fifth through seventh spots were also tied with a score of 199-15X. Clyde Brummet of Wolf City, TX, took fifth place over Rod Guthier, from Bloomington, MN, who had a "200" match going until he broke concentration on his very last shot. Guerry Dalrymple of Phoenix, AZ, was another example of determination as the configuration of his power wheelchair did not permit him a good position at the shooting table, and he had to transfer onto a small folding chair to shoot his medal winning score.

The eighth ranked competitor had never fired a gun before, but brought to the line a set of refined motor-control and concentration skills honed on her hobby of photography. Loretta Verbout from Rochester, MN, took home a medal as a result of shooting a fine score of 199-14X. It was quite evident by Loretta's performance of how similar the eye-hand coordination of a photographer is to that of a shooter.

Ninth place went to the 199-14X of Mike Kelly. Mike's fine shooting gave the Kelly family its second medal to take back home to Birmingham, as wife Hope had already claimed the gold medal.

The tenth and final NRA Medal was won by an outstanding performance turned in by Doug Bermel of Minneapolis, MN. Doug fired his 199-13X in a heavy wind that was actually blowing the target carrier back and forth. His match had to be interrupted while officials went downrange to add a large quantity of duct tape and a stabilizer bar to the target carrier. Doug was able to put these distractions aside and shoot a fine score.

None of the competitors realized it at the time, but they were all part of a history making event. This match had the highest number of disabled competitors to ever participate in a combined (able-bodied and disabled) .22 shooting competition in the United States. There were no special categories or classes, as everyone competed for the same medals on an equal basis with the result that seven of the top ten positions were won by shooters with disabilities.

This NRA Disabled Shooting Services designed match went a long way in demonstrating to the assembled officials of government agencies that shooting is truly an equal opportunity sports and recreation activity in which Americans with physical disabilities can participate in a safe and competent matter.

Directory of Clubs & Associations

The following organizations have as a goal *participation* in sport and recreational activities. For each organization, types of activities, events, competitions, publications, and contact information is provided where available. If funding or financial help is available, that is noted as well. Consult the *Index of Sports and Activities* to find all the organizations which have programs in your area of interest.

Achilles Track Club

One Times Square, 10th Floor
New York, NY 10036
Phone: 212/354-0300
Contact: Dick Traum

Description: Worldwide organization designed to encourage people with all kinds of disabilities to participate in long-distance running with the general public. While its activities focus in New York City, it has 111 chapters in 34 countries worldwide. There are 3,500 members.

Sports: Athletics, Long Distance Running, Quad Rugby, Shooting (Marksmanship), Swimming, Tennis, Wheelchair Basketball

Program/Services: Achilles Track Club coaches and trains wheelchair athletes to participate in marathon and other running events. Achilles focuses on the person who otherwise might not participate without help. ATC encourages people who want to run for pure enjoyment regardless of time, speed, and ability. Achilles has 25 spots in the NYC Marathon. A second area of activity is wheelchair basketball. Achilles sponsors a development wheelchair basketball league in the Bronx, consisting of 8 teams. Achilles Track Club is international in scope. Wheelchair athletes from Mongolia, Poland, South Africa, and New Zealand participate in Achilles events. Achilles introduced wheelchair participation in the Moscow Marathon.

Scholarships/Awards: Achilles holds a lottery to give away 5 racing wheelchairs among the finishers of the NYC Marathon.

Publications: Founder Dick Traum has written *A Victory for Humanity* with Mike Celizic (Waco,Tex.: WRS Publishing, 1993).

American Athletic Association for the Deaf (AAAD)

3607 Washington Blvd.
Suite 4
Ogden, UT 84403
Phone: 801/393-8710
TDD: TTY 801/393-7916
Fax: 801/393-2263
Contact: Shirley Platt, Executive Director

Description: AAAD is the national organization promoting sports and athletic competition for deaf athletes in the U.S. AAAD coordinates the participation of U.S. teams in international competition such as the World Games as well as regulates uniform rules of competition. Activities include annual children's sports festivals.

Sports: Alpine Skiing, Badminton, Baseball, Basketball, Bowling, Children/Youth Programs, Cycling, Flag Football, Golf, Ice Hockey, Nordic Snow Skiing, Orienteering, Shooting (Marksmanship), Soccer, Softball, Speed Skating, Swimming, Table Tennis, Team Handball, Tennis, Volleyball (Standing), Waterpolo, Wrestling

Manuals/Other Publications: *AAAD Bulletin; Deaf Sports Review; Regional Directory*

American Blind Bowling Association

67 Bame Avenue
Buffalo, NY 14215
Phone: 716/836-1472
Contact: Ron Beverly

Description: Oversees blind bowling leagues and sponsors an annual tournament.

Sports: Blind Bowling

Manuals/Other Publications: Publishes *The Blind Bowler*

American Blind Skiing Foundation

610 South William Street
Mt. Prospect, IL 60056
Phone: 708/255-1739

Description: A division of the United States Association for Blind Athletes. Volunteers teach downhill and cross-country skiing to persons with visual impairments.

Sports: Cross Country, Snow Skiing

Competition Events: Sponsors races and trips to skiing areas in Colorado, Wisconsin, and Michigan. Sponsors international races.

American Canoe Association, Inc. (Kayaking/Disabled Paddlers Committee)

7432 Alban Station Blvd.
Suite B-226
Springfield, VA 22150-2311
Phone: 703/451-0141
Fax: 703/451-2245
Contact: Jeffrey Yeager, Executive Director

Description: Dedicated to promoting canoeing, kayaking, and other paddlesports as lifetime recreational activities. It is affiliated with the U.S. Canoe and Kayak Team. Total membership is around 35,000.

Sports: Canoeing, Kayaking

Activities Offered: Conservation and River Access, Paddler Education Programs for the Physically and Economically Disadvantaged, ACA Canoe Safety Patrol Instruction, Athletic Competition, Touring.

Program/Services: Conducts national and international programs in safety, education, instruction, and competition, and promotes the sound use of the nation's recreational waterways through conservation and access programs.

Manuals/Other Publications: *Canoeing and Kayaking for Persons with Physical Disabilities Instruction Manual,* 1990, Anne Wortham Webre and Janet Zeller. One of a series of ACA instruction manuals, this book explores methods of instruction and of equipment modification for the physically challenged. Intended for instructors wishing to expand their skills, the manual assumes a basic knowledge of paddling. $14.95 (10% member discount).

Equipment: *Canoeing and Kayaking for Persons with Disabilities* lists adaptations for many specific disabilities and difficulties encountered by physically challenged canoers and kayakers.

American Sledge Hockey Association

10933 Johnson Ave. S
Bloomington, MN 55437-2911
Phone: 612/881-2129
Contact: John Schatzlein

Description: Sledge hockey is an exciting alternative winter sport that uses the rules of hockey. However, instead of skating, players sit on a specially designed sled and use two short ice picks to propel themselves across the ice. Standard hockey rules apply. Legal body contact and raised puck shooting are as much a part of sledge hockey as they are in stand-up hockey. The American Sledge Hockey Association was started in Minnesota with support from Canada, Great Britain, Sweden, and Norway. ASHA serves to provide assistance in team development and player skill development and can provide information on where to purchase sledge hockey equipment. ASHA also has sledges and picks available for trial use. Players must provide their own gloves and protective equipment, including hockey helmet.

Sports: Sledge hockey

Equipment: A tubular framed sledge, about 1.5 meters (4-5 feet) long and approximately 3 inches off the ice, with two hockey skate blades mounted beneath the seat. A portion of the front frame rests on the ice and provides lateral stability. Straps around the ankles, knees and waist securely hold the player on the sledge. Two half meter (29 in.) long "ice picks" are used to propel the sledge. The picks are simply modified hockey sticks with 4-cm teeth attached to the bottom of the non-blade end. Leaning left or right while digging a pick into the ice turns the sledge. Players slide to a stop on one or both blades, like a skater. All players wear regular protective hockey equipment.

American Waterski Association/Disabled Ski Committee

799 Overlook Dr.
Winter Haven, FL 33884
Phone: 813/324-4341
Contact: Leona Perry

Description: National Governing Body for Waterskiing that has a disabled sport division. Governs sport and sanctions events. Disabled skiers compete in slalom, tricks & jumping; rules are slightly different for disabled in terms of heights of ramps and other technical differences. Organization in existence since 1939; 30,000 members (able-bodied and disabled). There is a membership fee of $20 (supporting member) or $40 (competing member).

Sports: Waterskiing

Competition Events: National championships held in August each year (1995 Championships Aug. 18-20 in Elk Grove, CA)

Manuals/Other Publications: *The Waterskier,* 7 times yearly

Equipment: Multiplegics use a sit-ski; for tricking, a knee-board with a seat is used. Amputees use a regular slalom ski.

American Wheelchair Bowling Association

3620 Tamarack Drive
Redding, CA 96003
Phone: 916/243-2695
Fax: 916/243-2695
Contact: Walter Roy,
Executive Secretary-Treasurer

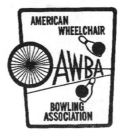

Description: The AWBA is a non-profit organization, formed in 1962, composed of wheelchair bowlers, dedicated to the encouragement, development and regulation of wheelchair bowling under uniform rules and regulations. The AWBA bowls under ABC (American Bowling Congress) Rules & Regulations or AWBA Rules, as adapted for wheelchair bowling. Promotes wheelchair bowling and sets playing rules. Maintains a hall of fame and museum.

Sports: Wheelchair Bowling

How to Start a Chapter: Contact your local bowling lanes for assistance. They can tell you what leagues you can join under ABC or WIBC rules. If you are unable to join an existing league, you may form your own wheelchair league by following the AWBA "Suggested League Rules" which can be obtained from the Association. It is recommended all leagues obtain ABC and WIBC sanctioning.

Competition Events: AWBA national tournaments are held each year. The climax of the bowling year, they are held in various areas of the country each year on a rotating basis. AWBA uses ABC year-end averages as the entering averages for the national tournaments. Any wheelchair bowler may qualify to bowl in a national tournament by bowling in an ABC sanctioned winter-league (21 game minimum) and holding valid AWBA and ABC memberships. Winter leagues generally start in September and bowl for 26 to 32 weeks (split season allowed). If league time is not available during the evening hours, it is best to schedule a league late in the afternoon (3 p.m.) or on weekends. Work with the lane management to have portable ramps available to get off the approaches and into the pit area while waiting to bowl.

Manuals/Other Publications: *Wheelchair Bowling* by Jim Lane, a wheelchair bowler for over 20 years ($10.00) may be purchased directly from the organization. AWBA publishes *The Eleventh Frame: A National Newsletter.*

Equipment: Bowling Ball Holder Ring, Ball Pusher, Handle Grip Bowling Ball, Bowling Ball Ramp

American Wheelchair Table Tennis Association

23 Parker Street
Port Chester, NY 10573
Phone: 914/835-3506
Contact: Jennifer Johnson, Associate Editor

Description: Promotes, initiates, and stimulates the growth and development of wheelchair and stand-up table tennis for the disabled in the United States. Group E member of the U.S. Olympic Committee. Has worked with U.S. Table Tennis Association. Affiliated with Wheelchair Sports, USA

Sports: Wheelchair Table Tennis

Competition Events: Members participate in Elite Athletes Training Camp; World Wheelchair Invitational Championship; the Paralympic Games; Irish National Championships; the U.S. Wheelchair National Table Tennis championships.

Manuals/Other Publications: *American Wheelchair Table Tennis Association Newsletter,* biannual

Amputees in Motion (AIM)

P.O. Box 2703
Escondido, CA 92033
Phone: 619/454-9300
Contact: William Handler,
President

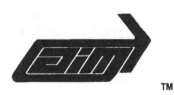

TM

Description: Amputees in Motion—for Fun! is a group of amputees organized in San Diego County in 1973 which offers counseling, encouragement, coaching, and role model leadership to amputees to engage in sports and recreation within the limitations posed by the type of amputation. Efforts are made to match the counselor to the type of amputee by age, sex, and type of amputation. AIM sponsors social activities, dinners, dances, picnics, sports, and similar events.
Sports: Archery, Bowling, General Recreation, Golf, Horseback

Sports, Everyone!
Riding, Snow Skiing, Waterskiing

Program/Services: Recreational or social events are planned monthly plus general meetings every two months. Activities, designed for both the amputee and family, include nonstrenuous sports, family events, and group sports. Programs include training persons to teach sports and to arrange recreational events. Areas covered include information on driving attachments, home aid, funding, license plates, education, and sports equipment.

ASPIRE (Association of Special People Inspired to Riding)

RD 4, Box 115
Malvern, PA 19355
Phone: 215/644-1963
Contact: Dottie Hefner, Executive Officer

Description: ASPIRE is a program at Thorncroft Equestrian Center in which disabled individuals are given the opportunity to ride and compete, win awards and ribbons. It is affiliated with North American Riding for Handicapped.

Sports: Horseback Riding

Scholarships/Awards: Scholarship to Thorncroft Center is given, based on need.

Manuals/Other Publications: Publishes a newsletter

BOLD—Blind Outdoor Leisure Development

Amanda C. Boxtel
P.O. Box 5266
Snowmass Village, CO 81615
Phone: 303/923-3871

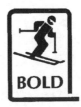

Description: BOLD of Aspen, Colorado, hosts legally blind skiers, providing instruction, blind skier guides, lodging at reasonable rates, and companions for shopping, driving, and other activities. BOLD can arrange transportation as well as provide equipment rental and certified blind ski guides who supervise and direct your skiing activities at all times.

Sports: Snow Skiing

Program/Services: The skiing season runs from Thanksgiving through April. Between Thanksgiving and Christmas and the first 2 weeks of April provide the best opportunity for reduced lodge rates and free ski instruction. Skating and snowmobiling can be arranged as well. In the summer season hiking, golfing, river-rafting, jeep tournaments, swimming, riding, and picnicking are all available and BOLD can help provide guides. There is also a very popular Braille Nature Trail in one of the accessible mountain areas.

Organization Slogan:
"When I ski, I'm free
I feel the wind in my face.
I fight the bumps with my legs.
For a minute I think I can see again."
—Jean Eymere, Founder

Boy Scouts of America

1325 W. Walnut Lane
Irving, TX 75038
Phone: 214/580-2000

Description: Scouting for the Handicapped Service is handled at the local troop level. Today more than 100,000 Cub Scouts, Boy Scouts, and Explorers with disabilities are registered with the Boy Scouts of America in more than 4,000 units that are chartered to community organizations. The basic premise of Scouting for people with special needs is that youth with disabilities want most to participate like other youth—and Scouting offers that chance. Thus, much of the program for Scouts with disabilities is directed at 1) helping unit leaders develop an awareness of the disabled among youth without disabilities, and 2) encouraging their inclusion in the regular Cub Scout pack, Boy Scout troop, Varsity Scout team, or Explorer post or ship. There are many units, however, composed of members with identical disabilities—an all-blind Boy Scout troop, an all-deaf Cub Scout pack, etc.—but these disabled members are encouraged to participate in Scouting activities along with nondisabled Scouts. Many of these special Scouting units are located in special schools or centers that make the Scouting program part of their curriculum.

Sports: Camping; General Sports

Program/Services: While the BSA's policy has always been to treat members with disabilities as much like other members as possible, it has been traditional to make some accommodations in advancement requirements if necessary. A Scout with a permanent physical or mental disability may apply to earn an alternate merit badge in lieu of a required badge, if the disabling condition prohibits the Scout from completing the necessary requirements of a particular badge. The policy is designed to keep Scouts with disabilities as much in the mainstream of Scouting as possible. Some of the National projects supported by the BSA include the Woods Services National Award for leaders in Scouting for the disabled; inclusion of materials relating to the disabled in the National Camping School syllabi; production of a new manual for individuals who are hearing impaired with major assistance from Gallaudet University; assignment of experienced staff.

Competition Events: An interpreter strip for Signing for the Deaf can be earned by all Scouts.

Manuals/Other Publications: Several publications are published by the BSA: *Scouting for the Physically Handicapped* (revised 1994); *Scouting for the Hearing Impaired* (revised 1990); *Scouting for the Blind and Visually Impaired* (revised 1990); and *Camp Directors Primer to the Americans with Disabilities Act of 1990* (1992).

Breckenridge Outdoor Education Center Activity

P.O. Box 697
Breckenridge, CO 80424
Phone: 303/453-6422
Contact: Lisa Reed

Description: Focus is on outdoor recreation including pure recreation, adventure therapy, and disability awareness.

Sports: Wilderness, Snow Skiing, Rock Climbing, Ropes Courses, rafting, Canoeing, Hiking, Camping

Program/Services: 1) Adaptive Ski Program; 2) Wilderness Programs, including rock climbing and high and low ropes courses (both of which are wheelchair accessible), rafting, canoeing, hiking, and camping; 3) Professional Challenge Program, group activities for team building

Organization Mission: To provide outdoor recreation for people of all abilities including mental and physical disabilities.

Canadian Association for Disabled Skiing (CANADA)

Box 307
Kimberly, BC V1A 2Y9
Phone: 604/427-7712
Fax: 604/427-7715
Contact: Jerry Johnston

Description: Nonprofit organization that sponsors skiing for the disabled of all ages. Divisions in each Canadian province except Prince Edward Island. Affiliated with Canadian Ski Association.

Sports: Alpine Skiing, Cross Country Skiing, Waterskiing (Alberta only)

Competition Events: National championships in spring. Location based on availability and conditions, date depends on location, though they try to coincide with the US nationals in Breckenridge.

Workshops: Ski instructor certification program

Publications: 2 newsletters per year

Canadian Wheelchair Sports Association/ Association Canadienne Des Sports En Fauteuil Roulant

1600 James Naismith Dr.
Gloucester, ON K1B 5N4
Phone: 613/748-5685
Fax: 613/748-5722

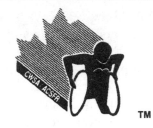

Description: Canada's development of wheelchair sports began in 1947. The Canadian Wheelchair Sports Association (CWSA) was officially formed in 1967 in Winnipeg, Manitoba, as a result of the organization for the Pan-Am Games. CWSA governs athletics, rugby, and tennis and supports the development of archery, basketball, racquetball, shooting, and swimming. Nationally, CWSA has 10 provincial associations which are responsible for conducting competitions and recreational programs to meet the needs of wheelchair athletes in each region. CWSA, as a volunteer, not-for-profit organization, operates on an annual budget of over three quarters of a million dollars. 40% is a combination of corporate sponsorship, donations and fundraising activity. Some of the facts about wheelchair sports and wheelchair athletes published by CWSA include: there are approximately 5,000 people participating in wheelchair sports in Canada. The most popular sport is wheelchair basketball, with over 2,000 Canadians playing in leagues around the country. Approximately 500 of these people are able-bodied participants. Wheelchair track is included in Athletics Canada's (able-bodied) junior and senior outdoor championships as full medal events. CWSA is committed to sports equity—providing opportunity for all Canadians without discrimination, to be treated fairly and equally in sport. There are approximately 3,000 members.

Sports: Archery, Athletics, Quad Rugby, Road Racing, Shooting (Marksmanship), Swimming, Track & Field, Wheelchair Basketball, Wheelchair Racquetball, Wheelchair Tennis

Scholarships/Awards: Application procedures are specified for particular grants.

Competition Events: Canada's technical programs develop athletes and teams who represent the country nationally and internationally against the best in the world. The Canadian Team consistently ranks in the top 5 internationally.

Manuals/Other Publications: *Communiqué,* a Newsletter

Casa Colina/Work It Out Program

2850 North Garey Ave.
Pomona, CA 91767
Phone: 909/596-7733
TDD: 909/596-3646
Fax: 909/596-7845
Contact: Ruth Shaeffer

Description: Casa Colina Centers for Rehabilitation are non-profit, community governed organizations which are internationally recognized leaders and innovators in the field of rehabilitation. Casa Colina's Outdoor Adventures is a unique program to empower people with disabilities by creating opportunities for challenging and exciting experiences in the out-of-doors. By focusing on abilities, not disabilities, the program enables its members to experience success both physically and emotionally. These adventures change lives. Through these activities people with disabilities can reaffirm belief in themselves and in their abilities to set new goals for a lifetime of achievement. Affiliated with Casa Colina Hospital for Rehabilitative Medicine.

Sports: Weight Training, Ocean Sailing, Rock Climbing, Whitewater Rafting, Snow Skiing, Horse Packing, Water Skiing, Deep Sea Fishing, Back Packing, Freshwater Fishing, Winter Camping, Dog Sledding, Sea Kayaking, and Family Camping.

Challenge Air for Kids and Friends

12728 Sunlight Dr.
Dallas, TX 75230
Phone: 214/701-0456
Contact: Rick Amber

Description: Nonprofit organization intended to provide recreational therapeutic flight to the disabled, usually in groups of 20-30. Rick

Amber is a certified flight instructor who also teaches flying to the disabled.

Activities Offered: Recreational therapeutic flight

Organization Slogan: The sky's the limit.

Cooperative Wilderness Handicapped Outdoor Group (C.W. Hog)

Idaho State University
Box 8118, Pond Student Union
Pocatello, ID 83209
Phone: 208/236-3912
Contact: Jeff Brandt

Description: Nonprofit group connected with Idaho State University that sponsors trips and other activities for the disabled. Trips are based on "common adventure" principle. Participants can receive academic credit for some of the activities. Organization is a "community self-help" model; instructors are volunteers.

Sports: Wilderness, Adaptive Swimming, Water Skiing, Snow Skiing, Weight Training, Whitewater Rafting, Rock Climbing, Scuba Diving, Skydiving, Dogsledding, Camping, Hiking, Fishing, Kayaking, Sailing, Pheasant Hunting, and Riding All-Terrain Vehicles.

Scholarships/Awards: There is a scholarship fund used to help defray the costs of trips for those with financial need.

Workshops: Whitewater rafting, water skiing, and snow skiing instruction workshops—for able-bodied who wish to teach these activities.

Disabled Sports USA

451 Hungerford Dr.
Suite 100
Rockville, MD 52246
Phone: 301/217-0960
Fax: 301/217-0968
Contact: Kirk M. Bauer, Executive Director

Description: Founded in 1967 by disabled Vietnam veterans, Disabled Sports USA is a national, non-profit organization providing year-round sports and recreational services to children and adults with disabilities. It serves over 30,000 annually through its national network of community-based chapters, and is a member of the U.S. Olympic Committee. It serves individuals with the following disabilities: physical disabilities which restrict mobility, including amputations, paraplegia, quadriplegia, cerebral palsy, head injury, multiple sclerosis, muscular dystrophy, spina bifida, stroke, and visual impairments. Disabled Sports USA has 87 community-based chapters in 40 states. Each chapter has its own individual programs and activities. (See article on page 15.)

Sports: Alpine Skiing, Archery, Cycling, Lawn Bowling, Nordic Snow Skiing, Powerlifting, Sailing, Swimming, Table Tennis, Volleyball (Sitting), Volleyball (Standing)

Program/Services: Winter Recreational Programs: Almost anyone with a physical disability can learn to ski. Each winter, Disabled Sports conducts the SKI SPECTACULAR for Disabled Skiers and numerous Learn to Ski, Learn to Race, and Learn to Teach clinics nationwide. Many chapters also conduct recreational ski programs. Disabled Sports conducts training camps for novices and advanced athletes in the sports listed above.

Organization Slogan: "If I can do this, I can do anything."

Competition Events: Disabled Sports conducts a series of Regional Ski Races that are qualifiers for the US Disabled Ski Championships. Level I races are for beginners to intermediate racers, Level II are for more advanced ski racers. Summer and Winter Competition Programs: Under the authority of the US Olympic Committee, Disabled Sports sanctions and conducts winter and summer competition in the sports listed above. In addition, Disabled Sports coordinates the US Disabled

51

Volleyball Team, a national team comprised entirely of ambulatory (standing) disabled athletes and the Alpine Junior Elite Team, the national's top junior disabled ski racers, ranging in age from 12-17.

Tapes/Videos: *Fitness is for Everyone* Videotapes (Exercise Programs); *Adaptive Ski Teaching Methods* Videotapes; *Children with Disabilities in Physical Education: Learning through Movement—A Parent Training Program; What is National Handicapped Sports*

Manuals/Other Publications: *Fitness Programming and Physical Disability; Children with Disabilities in Physical Education: Learning through Movement—a Parent Training Program*

How to Get Involved: To become a Disabled Sports competitive athlete, join your local chapter or be an at-large member. Participate in competitions and/or training camps; compete in local nondisabled events and forward your results to the Disabled Sports Competition Services Department. But remember, fitness is not just for the elite athlete. The passage of the Americans with Disabilities Act (ADA) mandates that properly adapted fitness programs become more widely available in community and rehabilitation centers. Additionally, disabled children are entitled to a proper adapted physical education in their public schools. Disabled Sports has videotapes and handbooks on these subjects.

Sponsors: An **Athlete Account** allows the athlete to raise and accept funds to cover training costs. It also entitles the donors to tax deductions for these gifts. Disabled Sports athletes who compete/train on a regional or national level are eligible to open Athlete Accounts. Organizations likely to give to a worthy cause include Chambers of Commerce; Church Groups; Kiwanis Clubs; Shriners; United Cerebral Palsy Assn.; Exercise Equipment Stores; Vietnam Veterans of America; Independent Living Centers; Optimists Clubs; Lions Clubs; Knights of Columbus; Easter Seals Societies; Spina Bifida Assn.; Athlete Shoe Stores; Disabled American Veterans Chapters; and your own family and friends. You should start your fund raising 6 months to 1 year ahead of time. Have a clear objective and a demonstrable budget. Learn about the organization you are approaching and look for a fit. Do it in person. Face-to-face meetings are far more effective in obtaining funding than written proposals alone, or even telephone communications. So call the individual in charge of bequests and ask for an appointment.

CHAPTERS

A.S.P.I.R.E. - Glenville
123 Saratoga Rd.
Glenville, NY 12302
Phone: (518) 437-9416
Contact: William Sampson

Adaptive Sports & Recreation of Topeka
2501 SE Michigan
Topeka, KS 66605
Phone: (913) 233-1961
Contact: Andy Hanschu

Adolescent Sarcoma Patients' Intensive Rehab. with Exercise
196 East 75th St.
New York, NY 10021
Phone: (212) 639-6713
Contact: Paddy Rossbach

Alabama Handicapped Sportsmen
11802 Creighton Ave.
Northport, AL 35476
Phone: (205) 339-2800
Contact: David Sullivan

Alpine Alternatives
2518 East Tudor Rd.
Suite 105
Anchorage, AK 99507
Phone: (907) 561-6655
Contact: Margaret Weber

American Sledge Hockey Assoc.
10933 Johnson Ave. South
Bloomington, MN 55437

Phone: (612) 881-2129
Contact: John Schatzlein

Aspen Handicapped Skiers Assoc.
PO Box 5429
Snowmass Village, CO 81615
Phone: (303) 923-3294
Contact: Edwin Lucks

Atlanta Chapter NHS
PO Box 327
Clarkston, GA 30021
Phone: (404) 498-7204
Contact: Stacy McPherson

Baltimore Adaptive Recreational Sports
301 Washington Ave.
Towson, MD 21204
Phone: (410) 887-5370
Contact: Pamela Harris-Lehnert

Beyond Barriers
1900 Brooks, Suite 115
Missoula, MT 59801
Phone: (406) 549-9878
Contact: Mike & Beth Manthey

Breckenridge Outdoor Educ. Center
PO Box 697
Breckenridge, CO 80424
Phone: (303) 453-6422
Contact: Rich Cook

California Handicapped Skiers
PO Box 2897
Big Bear Lake, CA 92315-2897
Phone: (714) 585-2519
Contact: Kelle Malkewitz, RTR

Cannonsburg Challenged Ski Assoc.
10831 Grange N.E.
Sparta, MI 49345-9451
Phone: (616) 887-4905
Contact: Kathy Fisher

Challenge Alaska
PO Box 110065
Anchorage, AK 99511-0065
Phone: (907) 563-2658
Contact: Patrick Reinhart

Challenge New Mexico
1570 Pacheco St. #E-6
Santa Fe, NM 87505
Phone: (505) 988-7621
Contact: Jane Hajovsky

Chesapeake Region Accessible Boating
PO Box 6564
Annapolis, MD 21401-0564
Phone: (410) 974-2628
Contact: Don Backe

Chicagoland Handicapped Skiers
1086 Briarcliffe
Wheaton, IL 60187
Phone: (708) 682-4018
Contact: Bud Sanders

Colorado Discover Ability
PO Box 3444

Grand Junction, CO 81502
Phone: (303) 242-0731
Contact: Pat White

Community Boating, Inc.
21 Embankment Rd.
Boston, MA 02114
Phone: (617) 523-1038
Contact: Bill Pendleton

Connecticut Handicapped Ski Foundation
PO Box 1805
Manchester, CT 06045-1805
Phone: (203) 645-0565
Contact: Maurice Collin

Courage Alpine Skiers
3915 Golden Valley Rd.
Golden Valley, MN 55422
Phone: (612) 520-0495
Contact: Kristi Youngguist

Courage Center
Twin Port Flyers
205 W. 2nd Street #451
Duluth, MN 55802
Phone: (218) 727-6874
Contact: Tim Kline

Courageous Sailing Center
1 First Ave, Charleston Navy Yd
Parris Building
Charleston, MA 02129
Phone: (617) 725-3263
Contact: Dru Slattery

Crested Butte Physically Challenged Skier Program
PO Box 5117
Mt. Crested Butte, CO 81225

Phone: (303) 349-2296
Contact: Carla Fanciullo

Deutsch Institute
615 Jefferson Ave, #201
Scranton, PA 18510
Phone: (717) 348-1968
Contact: Deborah Moran

Disabled Ski Prog. at Ski Windham
EPSIA Educational Foundation
1-A Lincoln Ave.
Albany, NY 12205-4900
Phone: (518) 452-6095
Contact: Gwen Allard

Disabled Sports Assoc. Of N. Texas
3810 W. Northwest High., Suite 205
Dallas, TX 75220
Phone: (214) 352-4100
Contact: Jerry McCole

Dream Disabled Ski Program
PO Box 8300
Kalispell, MT 59904-1300
Phone: (406) 758-5411
Contact: Sandy Center

Durango/Purgatory Adaptive Sports Association
PO Box 1884
Durango, CO 81301
Phone: (303) 259-0374
Contact: Susan Kroes

Eldora Special Recreation Program
PO Box 19016

Boulder, CO 80308-9016
Phone: (303) 442-0606
Contact: Sharon Kaylor

Footloose Sailing Assoc.
2319 N. 45th St., # 142
Seattle, WA 98103
Phone: (206) 632-3622
Contact: Karen Brattmayer

Front Range Sports
5556 Wheeling St.
Denver, CO 80239
Phone: (303) 966-5954
Contact: Nick Espinoza

Gaylord Hospital
PO Box 400
Wallingford, CT 06492
Phone: (203) 284-2800
Contact: Ken Murphy

Golf 4 Fun
PO Box 5304
Englewood, CO 80155
Phone: (303) 985-3403
Contact: Bob Nelson

Great Lakes Sailing Association for the Physically Disabled
150 West Jefferson, Suite 900
Detroit, MI 48220
Phone: (313) 255-7067
Contact: Dan Rustman

Greek Peak Sports for the Disabled
508 Verna Dr.
Endwell, NY 13760
Phone: (607) 785-6960
Contact: Dick Wierman

Houston Area Chapter, NOAP
11603 Orchard Mountain Dr.
Houston, TX 77059
Phone: (713) 334-1993
Contact: Larry Smith

Hunter Mt. Disabled Ski Program
PO Box 433
Hunter, NY 12442
Phone: (518) 263-4278
Contact: David Chaffee

I Am Third Foundation dba Eagle Mount - Billings
PO Box 20233
Billings, MT 59104
Phone: (406) 245-5422
Contact: Debra Speer

I Am Third Foundation dba Eagle Mount - Great Falls
4237 2nd Avenue North
Great Falls, MT 59401
Phone: (406) 454-1449
Contact: Marion Gutzwiler

I Am Third Foundation-Eagle Mount
6901 Goldenstein Lane
Bozeman, MT 59715
Phone: (406) 586-1781
Contact: Art Lawson

Jed Goldman Adaptive Sailing Prg.
425 East McFetridge Dr.
Chicago, IL 60605
Phone: (312) 294-2270
Contact: Ted Sutherland

Lakeside Chapter NHS
749 Veterans Memorial Dr.
Las Vegas, NV 89101
Phone: (702) 229-6297
Contact: John Chambers

Loon Mountain NHS
55 Washington Ave.
Boston, MA 02152
Phone: (603) 745-8111
Contact: Robert Harney, M.D.

Lounsbury Ski Program
PO Box 370
Ellicottville, NY 14731
Phone: (716) 699-2345
Contact: Jane Probst

Maine Handicapped Skiing
Sunday River Ski Resort
RR2, Box 1971
Bethel, ME 04217-9600
Phone: (207) 824-2440
Contact: Paula Wheeler

Mesa Association of Sports for the Disabled
PO Box 4727
Mesa, AZ 85211-4727
Phone: (602) 649-2194
Contact: Gregg Baumgarten

Michigan Handicapped Sports & Recreation Assoc.
238 Woodview Ct. Apt 244
Rochester Hills, MI 48307-4191
Phone: (313) 853-0648
Contact: Lee Helms

Mother Lode Chapter
PO Box 4274
Camp Connell, CA 95223
Phone: (909) 795-5811
Contact: Richard K. Van Aken

Nat. Sports Ctr. for the Disabled
PO Box 36
Winter Park, CO 80482
Phone: (303) 726-5514
Contact: Paul Dibello

Nation's Capital Handicapped Sports
PO Box 220254
Chantilly, VA 22022-0254
Phone: (202) 234-6275
Contact: Lina Padilla

National Ability Center
PO Box 682799
Park City, UT 84068
Phone: (801) 649-3991
Contact: Meeche White

National Amputee Summer Sports Assoc., Ltd.
215 West 92nd St., Suite 15A
New York, NY 10025
Phone: (212) 874-4138
Contact: Susan Ehrenfeld, R.N.

National Ocean Access Project
PO Box 10726
Rockville, MD 20849-0726
Phone: (301) 217-9843
Contact: Ed Harrison

New England Handicapped Sportsmen's Assoc.
26 McFarlin Rd.
Chelmsford, MA 01824
Phone: (508) 256-3240
Contact: Earl Plummer

NHS of Orange County
22361 Pine Glen
Mission Viejo, CA 92692
Phone: (714) 586-7754
Contact: Robert Mitchell

NHS of Southern California "The Unrecables"
PO Box 24856
Los Angeles, CA 90024
Phone: (310) 374-6775
Contact: Linda Fryback

Northeast Passage
PO Box 127
Durham, NH 03824-0127
Phone: (603) 862-0070
Contact: Jill Gravnick

Northern California Chapter NHS
6060 Sunrise Vista Dr., #3030
Citrus Heights, CA 95610
Phone: (916) 722-6447
Contact: Douglas J. Pringle

Northern California Chapter NHS-Tahoe Adaptive Ski
PO Box 9780
Truckee, CA 95737
Phone: (916) 581-4161
Contact: Katherine Hayes

Operation Able/Sail
PO Box 842
Moncton, NB E1C 8H7
Phone: (506) 857-3988
Contact: Michael Dunn

**Paraplegics on Independent
Nature Trips (P.O.I.N.T)**
4144 North Central Expwy, #515
Dallas, TX 75204
Phone: (214) 827-7404
Contact: Jules Brenner

**Philadelphia Area Handi-
capped Skiing Club**
4318 Spruce St.
Philadelphia, PA 19003
Phone: (215) 222-6277
Contact: Isabel Bohn

**Physically Adapted Recr. &
Sports**
c/o Memorial Regional Rehab.
Ctr.
PO Box 16406
Jacksonville, FL 32245-6406
Phone: (904) 399-6884
Contact: Janet Collins

Recreation Unlimited, Inc.
PO Box 447
Boise, ID 83701
Phone: (208) 336-3293
Contact: Van Tran

RIC-Skiers
Rehab. Institute of Chicago
345 E. Superior St.
Chicago, IL 60611
Phone: (312) 908-4292
Contact: Jeff Jones

**Richmond Athletes with Dis-
abilities Sports**
PO Box 311
Richmond, VA 23202-9998
Phone: (804) 747-7769
Contact: Suzie Groach

**Rocky Mountain Handicapped
Sportsmen's Association**
PO Box 18036 Capital Hill Sta-
tion
Denver, CO 80218
Phone: (303) 934-9540
Contact: Tom Reetz

San Diego Adventurers
3169 Winlow St.
San Diego, CA 92105
Phone: (619) 582-3871
Contact: Charlene Rawls

Sea Legs
88 Kelvin Ave.
Staten Island, NY 10306
Phone: (718) 987-6837
Contact: Ken Craig

South Florida Chapter NHS
c/o Health South Sunrise Rehab.
Ft. Lauderdale, FL 33351
Phone: (305) 749-0300
Contact: Dave Rafter

**Southern Chesapeake Adap-
tive Maritime Program**
PO Box 62567
Virginia Beach, VA 23466
Phone: (804) 463-8649
Contact: Arn Manella

Southern Colorado Center for Challenged Athletes
1124 S. Russett Dr.
Pueblo West, CO 81007
Phone: (719) 547-2337
Contact: Royce A. Miller

Southwest Wheelchair Athletic Assoc
4144 N. Central Expressway, Suite 515
Dallas, TX 75205
Phone: (214) 828-1406
Contact: Judy Einbinder

Special Outdoor Leisure Opportunities, Inc.
PO Box 6221
South Bend, IN 46660
Phone: (219) 237-5252
Contact: Ellen & David Grinnell

Sports, Arts & Recr. of Chatta-nooga
Slaten's House of Wheelchairs
3230 Brainerd Rd.
Chattanooga, TN 37411
Phone: (615) 622-5172
Contact: Andy Lane

Sundown Handicapped Skiers
1341 Cummins Ct.
Dubuque, IA 52001
Phone: (319) 556-6676
Contact: Thomas Gavin

Team USAble
PO Box 4124
Bellingham, WA 98227
Phone: (206) 671-5771
Contact: Doug Mackey

The Adaptive Ski Program
2425 Ridgecrest Dr. SE
Albuquerque, MN 87108
Phone: (505) 262-7563
Contact: Ken Ley

Three Rivers Adaptive Sports
P.O. Box 38235
Pittsburgh, PA 15238
Phone: (412) 749-2281
Contact: Mark Kulzer

Three Trackers of Ohio
16815 Forestwood Dr.
Strongsville, OH 44136
Phone: (216) 238-1166
Contact: Kate Gordon

Utah Handicapped Skiers Assoc.
P.O. Box 543
Roy, UT 84067-0543
Phone: (801) 777-7029
Contact: Steve Peterson

Vermont Handicapped Ski & Sports Assoc.
PO Box 261
Brownsville, VT 05037
Phone: (802) 484-3525
Contact: Laura Farrell

Warriors on Wheels
409 Hackett Blvd.
Albany, NY 12208
Phone: (518) 453-9205
Contact: Ned Norton

Waterville Valley Disabled
Athletes Program
Waterville Valley, NH 03215
Phone: (603) 236-8311
Contact: Kathy Chandler

Fishing Has No Boundaries

P.O. Box 175
Hayward, WI 54843
Phone: 715/634-3185
Contact: Tom Mansfield, VP of Operations

Description: For the disabled of all ages. No limits on who may participate, no matter the age or disability. 8 chapters throughout U.S., 3
additional in '96, 2 in Canada. Nonprofit, all-volunteer organization.
Each chapter puts on annual 2- or 3-day event on water. Fee includes
meals, bait, boats, guides, fuel, tents, port-a-potties, etc. In existence
since 1986.

Sports: Fishing

CHAPTERS

Eagle River Event
P.O. Box 2200
Eagle River, WI 54521
Phone: 715/479-7735
Toll free: 800/261-FISH
Contact: Will Campbell

Hayward Event
P.O. Box 375
Hayward, WI 54843
Phone: 715/634-3185
Contact: Dan Paullin

Illinois
157 Hillcrest Ave.
Wood Dale, IL 60191

Phone: 312/481-0000
Contact: Ron Canova

Madison Event
4923 Hammersley Road
Madison, WI 53711
Phone: 608/271-0440
Contact: Bill Jansen

Minnesota
Bemidji Chamber of Commerce
300 Bemidji Ave. P.O. Box 850
Bemidji, MN 56601
Toll free: 800/458-2223
Contact: Carol Olson

Ohio
3807 Deerpath Drive
Sandusky, OH 44870
Phone: 419/626-6211
Contact: Ron Marvicsin

South Dakota
Pierre Area Chamber of Commerce
P.O. Box 548

Pierre, SD 57501
Toll free: 800/962-2034
Contact: Karen Kern

Wyoming
HSC Chamber of Commerce
250 Arapahoe St. Box 768
Thermopolis, WY 82443
Phone: 307/864-3192
Contact: Wayne Bentel

Freedom's Wings International

1832 Lake Ave.
Scotch Plains, NJ 07076
Phone: 908/232-6354
Contact: Raymond D. Temchus

Description: Freedom's Wings International is a non-profit, all volunteer, New Jersey-based organization run by and for people with physical disabilities. Freedom's Wings provides the opportunities for those who are physically challenged to fly in specially adapted sailplanes, either as a passenger, or as a member of the flight training program. The goal is to bring the experience of soaring to the physically challenged. An introductory flight generally lasts 20 minutes. An instructional flight, where pilot and student are working to gain altitude by riding rising thermal currents, may last as long as two hours. Operates from Van Sant Airport in Erwinna (Bucks Co.), PA. An introductory flight for a person with disabilities is free. Subsequent flights are $25.

Sports: Soaring

Program/Services: Flying sessions are scheduled 7 days/week, weather permitting. Currently operates 4 sail-planes in its entry-level and graduate flying program. These gliders are equipped with hand controls. Potential students are screened by flight instructors certified by the FAA. Students receive training using FAA-approved curriculum. The flying season runs from April 1 to December 1. Students from all over the country as well as international, have been hosted by club members. Special demonstrations are available. Sailplanes may be partially disassembled for easy transport in a special trailer.

Scholarships/Awards: A limited number of scholarships is available. Special fundraising events provide funds for scholarships and equipment maintenance.

Girl Scouts of the USA

420 5th Ave.
New York, NY 10018
Phone: 212/852-8000
Fax: 212/852-6515
Contact: Colleen Floyd

Description: Services for Girls with Disabilities are handled through referrals to local troops. Training for scout leaders.

Sports: Camping; General Sports

Publications: *Focus on Ability: Serving Girls with Special Needs,* by Mary E. Carroll, Ed.D., is a publication intended to introduce volunteer leaders to the subject of disabilities; how to introduce a disabled member to a troop; how to simulate disabilities in order to foster sensitivity to disabilities; and definitions of, classifications of, myths and stereotypes of, characteristics of, adaptations for, and famous people with seven different classifications of disabilities (visual disabilities, hearing disabilities, learning disabilities, communication disorders, mental retardation, behavior disorders, physical and health disabilities).

Handicapped Scuba Association (HSA International)

1104 El Prado
San Clemente, CA 92672-4637
Phone/Fax: 714/498-6128

Description: Founded in 1981 by Jim Gatacre, HSA International is a 501(c)3 non-profit corporation that is the world's leading authority on recreational diving for people with disabilities.
Sports: Scuba diving

Programs/Services: Operates as an independent diver training and certifying agency. Offers diver education programs and Instructor Training Course. "Dive Buddy Program" offers able-bodied divers the chance to dive with a disabled partner. Several leading rehabilitation hospitals in the U.S. have included HSA scuba classes as part of their out-patient programs. Affiliated with Professional Diving Instructors Association and National Association of Underwater Instructors.

Videos: *Freedom in Depth* ($35.00); *To Fly in Freedom* ($35.00).

International Wheelchair Aviators

1117 Rising Hill Way
Escondido, CA 92029
Phone: 619/746-5018

Description: Disseminates information about the ability of physically disabled persons to fly planes.

Sports: Flying

Competition Events: Sponsors monthly fly-ins.
Manuals/Other Publications: Publishes a monthly newsletter

International Wheelchair Road Racers Club

30 Myano Lane
Stamford, CT 06902
Phone: 203/967-2231
Fax: 203/327-7999
Contact: Joseph M. Dowling

Description: Former National Governing Body for wheelchair track & field; most of its duties have now been taken over by Wheelchair Athletics of the USA. Operates mainly as a type of watchdog organization. There are over 900 members.

Sports: Wheelchair Track & Field

Jumping Mouse Camp, Inc.

215 N. Bonito
Flagstaff, AZ 86001
Phone: 602/774-9608
Contact: Jeffe Aronson, Director

Description: Canoeing/rafting trips through the Grand Canyon area. No trips planned at present; will be out of the country until 2/96. Note: For a listing of Outfitters operating special population charter trips, call Park Service at 502/638-7701.

Sports: Canoeing, rafting

Manuals: *River Trips for People with Special Needs*

Videos: Hour-long documentary of first oar trip, shown nationally on PBS, $20.

National Amputee Golf Association (NAGA)

P.O. Box 1228
Amherst, NH 03031
Fax: 603/672-7140
Contact: Jim Coombes, Executive Director

Description: In 1954 this organization was founded by a small group of amputees who recognized the importance of their own participation in the sport of golf to their rehabilitation. Believing that what had worked for them could work for others, they founded NAGA. Supported by the PGA, the USGA, and the Disabled American Veterans Association, NAGA is over 3,000 members strong, with State and Regional affiliates.

Sports: Golf

Program/Services: NAGA's "1st Swing...Golf for the Physically Challenged program" is a program developed to instruct therapists to teach and encourage the physically challenged to learn or re-learn golf. It is offered free of cost to the hosting facility thanks to the sponsorship of the PGA and the DAV Charitable Trust. It is a 2-day seminar hosted by rehabilitation hospitals, parks, and recreation departments, and prosthetic concerns. Day 1 is a learning course on golf for the physically challenged. Day 2 is devoted to therapists under the tutelage of members of the NAGA's "1st Swing team." The program is open to every physically challenged person regardless of age or handicap. The program is approved for Continuing Education credit by the PGA. It is NAGA's hope that PGA professionals will attend seminars and learn how to adapt instruction to the needs of the physically challenged.

Scholarships/Awards: Offers college scholarships.

Organization Slogan: "Adopt a Hospital"

Competition Events: Sponsors local, regional, and national tournaments.
Manuals/Other Publications: Publishes *Amputee Golfer Magazine* (annual).

National Beep Baseball Association

2231 West First Avenue
Topeka, KS 66606-1304
Phone: 913/234-2156
Contact: Jeanette Bigger, Chairperson

Description: National Governing Body for Beep Baseball—governs and promotes the sport and sanctions tournaments and World Series. Beep Baseball is a form of baseball adapted for the visually impaired. A 16-inch electronic beeping softball is used, along with 4-ft-tall round, foam, buzzing bases. Of the nine players on each team, six must be visually impaired (they are blindfolded to ensure that no one has an unfair advantage) and three are sighted. 300-400 people and 17 teams are registered. Many more unregistered teams play. $25 team registration fee; individual is $5 before June 1, $10 after.

Sports: Beep Baseball

Competition Events: Regional tournaments and a World Series is played. Potential hosts for the World Series are encourage to apply two years ahead of time; they are in charge of running the event and bear most of the costs; the NBBA is there to help out and add some additional funding.

Workshops: The NBBA can put on workshops if help for a team is needed.

Manuals/Other Publications: Manuals on rules, refereeing, etc., are available. Information packet is available; newsletter 4 times a year.

Equipment: Beep baseballs and buzzing bases, built by the Telephone Pioneers of America

National Foundation of Wheelchair Tennis

940 Calle Amanecer
Suite B
San Clemente, CA 92673
Phone: 714/361-6811
Fax: 714/361-6822
Contact: Brad Parks

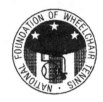

TM

Description: The National Governing Body for Wheelchair Tennis. Since its inception in 1976, wheelchair tennis has been the fastest growing of all wheelchair sports. The rules of wheelchair tennis follow those set forth by the International Tennis Federation with one major exception—the wheelchair player is allowed two bounces of the ball. The first bounce must be within the boundaries of the court, the second bounce may land anywhere. There are several men's and women's divisions in competitive wheelchair tennis ranging from Open (the most advanced players) to the D division for the novice player. There are junior divisions for players under 18 years of age and 2 quadriplegic divisions for those with upper extremity weakness. Participants from more than 30 nations actively participate in the sport. In 1989 the International Wheelchair Tennis Federation was formed to organize and promote the sport on an international basis. Regions are: New England (Maine, Rhode Island, Vermont, Massachusetts, Connecticut); Eastern (New York); Middle States (Pennsylvania, New Jersey, Delaware); Mid-Atlantic (Maryland, Virginia, West Virginia, DC); Southern (North Carolina, South Carolina, Tennessee, Arkansas, Louisiana, Mississippi, Alabama, Georgia); Florida; Caribbean (Puerto Rico, US Virgin Islands); Western (Wisconsin, Illinois, Indiana, Ohio, Michigan); Northwestern (North Dakota, South Dakota, Minnesota); Missouri Valley (Nebraska, Kansas, Oklahoma, Iowa, Missouri); Texas; Southwestern (Arizona, New Mexico); Intermountain (Montana, Wyoming, Idaho, Colorado, Utah, Nevada); USTA/Pacific Northwest (Oregon, Washington, British Columbia, Alaska); Northern California; Southern California. The Wheelchair Tennis Players Association (WTPA) was formed in 1981 under the auspices of the National Foundation. It was formed so that players could take an active role of the governance of their sport. WTPA fosters competitive wheelchair tennis throughout the world, establishes and enforces rules, organizes tournaments, and formulates a uniform ranking system. Affiliated with Wheelchair Sports USA.

Total Membership: 10,000+ (from age 7 and up)

Sports: Wheelchair Tennis

Program/Services: The Grand Prix circuit was created in 1981. In 1984 this became known as the Everest and Jennings Grand Prix Circuit. Since 1981, there has also been a great emphasis placed upon the development of programs for children. Junior programs include junior wheelchair sports camps programs, tennis training camps, and ongoing wheelchair tennis instruction.

Scholarships/Awards: Grants from the USTA (up to $500) have been made available for the implementation and support of wheelchair tennis programs. These funds are not available for tournament support. Regional sections have scholarships monies available for such activities as tennis camps.

Competition Events: There are 70 sanctioned tournaments nationally, culminating in October each year. This tournament is attended by wheelchair athletes from throughout the world. This tournament involves about 300 athletes in fierce competition. In a typical year, there are 8 tournaments throughout the US, 2 USTA National championships, 5 regional championship events, and the US Open Wheelchair Tennis Championships. This event has become known as the "Wimbledon of Wheelchair Tennis."

Tapes/Videos: Videos include: *Tennis in a Wheelchair* ($29.95); *Advanced Wheelchair Tennis* ($29.95); *Highlights of the 1990 U.S. Open* ($29.95); *More than Tennis* ($29.95); and *Sharing is Caring: Highlights of the Junior Wheelchair Sports Camp.* This camp serves as a model to parks and recreation departments throughout the nation. Narrated by Lloyd Bridges ($25).

Manuals/Other Publications: Manual: *Tennis in a Wheelchair: an instructional booklet on wheelchair tennis* ($7.50); Monthly Newsletter, *Two Bounce News* ($5.00/yr); *Sports Camp Guidelines* ($5.00); *WTPA Rules Booklet* ($6.00); plus packets: *Camp* ($5.00); *Instructional* ($40.00 -video included); and *Tournament* ($3.00).

Sponsors: The NFWT is funded through the philanthropic and the commercial sector of society with support coming from many fineorganizations, companies, and private individuals. Among the professional tennis players who have supported the organization are Ivan Lendl, Stefan Edberg, Pete Sampras, Rick Leach, Jim Pugh, John Fitzgerald, Sherwood Stewart, Danie Visser, and Pieter Aldrich.

National Library Service for the Blind and Physically Handicapped

Library of Congress
Washington D.C.,

Description: This large print series features free pamphlets on recreational activities for the physically challenged. The publications bring together resources in print, braille, cassettes, and reprints of diaries and other literature in order to introduce these activities and point the reader to further research. Publications in the series include: *Horses: An Introduction to Racing, Ranching, and Riding for Blind and Physically Handicapped Individuals; Birding: An Introduction to Ornithological Delights for Blind and Physically Handicapped Individuals; Sailing: An Introduction to the Wonders of Sailing for Blind and Physically Handicapped Individuals; Fishing: An Introduction to Fishing for Fun and Food for Blind and Physically Handicapped Individuals;* and *Swimming: An Introduction to Swimming, Diving, and SCUBA Diving for Blind and Physically Handicapped Individuals.*

Sports: Birding, Fishing, Horseback Riding, Sailing, Scuba Diving, Swimming

National Ocean Access Project

P.O. Box 33141
Farragut Station
Washington, DC 20033

Description: Develops and promotes marine-oriented recreational opportunities.

Sports: Canoeing, Kayaking, Rafting, Sailing

Competition Events: Sponsors a national regatta using boats designed for people with mobility impairments.

Manuals/Other Publications: Quarterly Newsletter, *Ocean Access*

National Skeet Shooting Association

P.O. Box 680007
San Antonio, TX 78268
Phone: 210/688-3371
Contact: Mary Masch, ext. 112

Description: National Governing Body for skeet shooting—governs the sport and sanctions events. The association has a wheelchair division that sponsors events that run concurrently with events for the able-bodied; a handicapped field with access for the disabled is available for these events. There are 756 different clubs and thousands of events taking place yearly across the country. Membership fee is $20. It is affiliated with National Sporting Clays.

Sports: Skeet Shooting

Publication: *Skeet Shooting Review,* monthly magazine

Equipment: No special equipment beyond a shotgun is needed, although some wheelchair shooters may make adaptations in their wheelchairs for greater mobility.

National Sports Center for the Disabled

P.O. Box 36
Winter Park, CO 80482
Phone: 303/726-5514

Description: Offers winter skiing and summer mountain recreation for the disabled. The NSCD is a non-profit corporation with an annual budget of $2.4 million. These funds are raised through program fees, corporations, foundations, special events, individual donations, planned giving, and generous in-kind donations from the Winter Park Resort. Staffed by volunteers. Affiliated with National Handicapped Sports.

Sports: Fishing, Hiking, Rock Climbing, Snow Skiing, Whitewater Rafting, Hiking, Camping, Mountain Biking, Hayrides, Ranch Trips, Fishing, and Alpine Slide Rides

Program/Services: Skiing 7 days a week, Dec. through April; Summer recreation program 4 days a week (Mon-Thurs) include whitewater rafting, hiking, and other mountain activities

Workshops: Over 800 skiing lessons taught each week

National Wheelchair Basketball Association

c/o Stan Labanowich
University of Kentucky
110 Seaton Building
Lexington, KY 40506
Phone: 909/596-7733
Fax: 606/258-1090
Contact: Stan Labanowich,
Commissioner

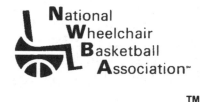

TM

Description: The NWBA was founded in 1949 in Galesburg, IL, at the conclusion of the First National Invitational Wheelchair Basketball Tournament. There were 6 charter teams from Kansas City, Hannibal, Evansville, Chicago, Minneapolis, and Illinois. The NWBA incorporated additional teams that had their origins in the Veteran Administration Hospitals and others from civic locations.Today there are well over 160 teams in the US and Canada, playing in 27 conferences and divisions. Teams vie annually for the opportunity to compete in post season tournament competition leading to the national championship. Wheelchair basketball is played according to NCAA rules with only a few modifications introduced to account for the use of the wheelchair. The dribble rule is different (accounting for the motion of the wheelchair) and, instead of a 3-second rule in the lane, a 4-second time limit is applied. Divisions include the Women's Division, Youth Division, NWBA Independents (non-conference affiliated) and 18 conferences.

Affiliated with Wheelchair Sports USA.

Sports: Wheelchair Basketball

Program/Services: Wheelchair basketball local, regional, and national play; camps (with PVA); Hall of Fame; awards.

Scholarships/Awards: Association with USA Basketball has freed the players on the national teams from having to raise funds for participation as a precondition of their participation.

Competition Events: Men: the NWBA provides for the annual determination of a national championship team through the establishment of a graduated post season competition involving regional and sectional tournaments in order to advance 4 teams to the national tournament which is conducted as a single elimination playoff similar to that of the NCAA. Women: A national tournament is held for women's teams and administered by the Women's Division of the NWBA. There are currently 11 women's teams in the Association although women are permitted to play on men's teams in areas where there are too few women to organize separately. Collegians: There have been 17 national tournaments for collegiate teams administered through the Central Intercollegiate Conference which is presently made up of 7 teams. Players are required to meet eligibility standards as outlined in their institutions' membership in the NCAA and NAIA. Juniors: Since 1993, 2 national championships for juniors have been held, the first involving 13 teams and the second 14 teams. Players are required to be 21 or younger.

Manuals/Other Publications: NWBA Newsletter; NWBA Directory;1994-95 Constitution Bylaws and Executive Regulations; NWBA Rules and Case Book.

How to Get Involved: There are teams all across the country. Contact the national office to find teams near you. The full roster of the NWBA may be found on page 177.

National Wheelchair Racquetball Association

Greater Pittsburgh Rehab Hospital
2380 McGinley Rd.
Monroeville, PA 15146
Phone: 412/856-2468
Contact: Geno Bonetti

Description: National Governing Body for Wheelchair Racquetball. In conjunction with AARA, help to govern and set up events and competitions for wheelchair racquetball; also some competitions between wheelchair and able-bodied racquetball players. It is affiliated with Wheelchair Sports USA; American Amateur Racquetball Association.

Sports: Wheelchair Racquetball

Competition Events: Number of competitions varies year to year, but normally about 20-25 in the US per year. Nationals take place in Houston.

Tapes/Videos: *Wheelchair Racquetball,* $45; sales are used as a fundraiser.

National Wheelchair Shooting Federation

102 Park Ave.
Rockledge, PA 19046
Phone: 703/267-1495
Contact: David Baskin

Description: National governing body for Wheelchair Shooting. The National Wheelchair Shooting Federation runs shooting events at regional competitions—there are about 20 such competitions around the country. Also trains disabled shooters and takes the US team overseas. It is affiliated with Wheelchair Sports, USA.

Sports: Shooting (Marksmanship)

Competition Events: Runs and governs shooting events at regional competitions.

National Wheelchair Softball Association

1616 Todd Ct.
Hastings, MN 55033
Phone: 612/437-1792
Contact: John Speake

Description: Referrals to local groups. 30 teams nationwide.

Sports: Wheelchair Softball

North American Riding for the Handicapped Association (NARHA)

P.O. Box 33150
Denver, CO 80233
Phone: 303/452-1212

Description: NARHA was formed for riders with disabilities. NARHA establishes safety standards, provides continuing education and offers networking opportunities for both its individual and operating center members. Therapeutic riding is recognized by the American Occupational Therapy Association and the American Physical Therapy Association. The benefits of therapeutic riding are available to individuals with just about any disability, including Muscular Dystrophy; Visual/ Hearing Impairments; Mental Retardation; Multiple Sclerosis; Emotional Disabilities; Spinal Cord Injuries; Learning Disabilities; Cerebral Palsy; Down Syndrome; Autism; Spina Bifida; Brain Injuries; Amputations; CVA/Stroke. Research shows that students who participate in therapeutic riding can experience physical, emotional, and mental rewards. For individuals with impaired mobility, horseback riding gently and rhythmically moves their bodies in a manner similar to human walking gait. These riders can experience increased balance, muscle control, and strength.

Sports: Horseback Riding, Instructional Training

Program/Services: Offers training and certification for riding instructors working with persons with disabilities. More than 450 member operating centers in the US and Canada, ranging from small, one-person programs to large operations with several instructors and therapists. In addition to therapeutic riding, an operating center may offer any number of equine activities for individuals with disabilities. Based on its qualifications, a center may offer driving, vaulting, hippotherapy, trail riding, competition, or stable management. More than 23,000 riders are served. Provides therapeutic classes using horseback riding to improve motor development and well-being of children and adults with physical and mental disabilities in accredited centers.

How to Start a Chapter: To start a program, NARHA offers a Start-Up Packet for $10. It includes information on personnel, facilities, insurance, funding, equipment, and sample forms.

Tapes/Videos: *NARHA Driving Video* ($22.50/nonmember $27.50); Promotional video ($20/nonmember $25)

Manuals/Other Publications: *NARHA General Workshop Notebook* ($30/nonmember $50); *NARHA Driving Handbook* ($5); *NARHA Curriculum for Riding Therapy* ($40/nonmember $65) Publishes a quarterly newsletter, *NARHA News*. The *NARHA Guide* is free with membership.

One-Arm Dove Hunt Association

Box 582
Olney, TX 76374
Phone: 817/564-2102

Description: Provides local shooting competitions for those with hand or arm amputations. Sponsors local competitions.

Sports: Shooting (Marksmanship)

Outdoors Forever

P.O. Box 4832
East Lansing, MI 48823
Phone: 517/337-0018
Contact: Don Basye

Description: A nonprofit organization begun in 1986 to promote outdoors recreation for the elderly and disabled, but also is an inclusive organization that welcomes able-bodied participants of all ages. The organization has worked as an advocate for the disabled by sitting on various committees in the state of Michigan (including 504 Transition and Implementation committees) and has worked to get various laws passed. Provide information free of charge on products for fishing, hunting, camping and other outdoors activities. It is affiliated with Michigan United Conservation and Michigan Nonprofit Forum.

Membership Fee: Fee for fishing tournament is set yearly.

Sports: Fishing

Organization Slogan: "Making the outdoors accessible for all." (registered)

Competition Events: Annual summer fishing tournament in Oscoda, MI (the location may change in the future), attracting approximately 125 participants

Workshops: Have sponsored workshops on accessibility.

Equipment: Sizable inventory of fishing, hunting, and outdoors-related equipment.

Outward Bound National Office

Route 9D
R-2 Box 280
Garrison, NY 10524-9757
Phone: 800/243-8520

Description: Outward Bound provides wilderness activities and programs. There are 5 wilderness schools (in Maine, North Carolina, Minnesota, Colorado, and Oregon) and programs in 22 states. All courses require a physical; approval is based on the results of the physical. While there are no specific programs for the disabled, many of the wilderness activities are suitable for persons with certain disabilities.

Sports: Wilderness Training

CHAPTERS

Colorado Outward Bound School
945 Pennsylvania St.
Denver, CO 80203-3198
Toll free: 800/477-2627

Hurricane Island Outward Bound School
PO Box 429
Rockland, ME 04841
Toll free: 800/341-1744

North Carolina Outward Bound School
121 North Sterling Street

Morganton, NC 28655-3443
Toll free: 800/841-0186

Pacific Crest Outward Bound School
0110
Portland, OR 97201
Toll free: 800/547-3312

Voyageur Outward Bound School
111 3rd Avenue S
Minneapolis, MN 55401-2551
Toll free: 800/328-2943

Paralyzed Veterans of America (PVA)

801 Eighteenth St. NW
Washington, DC 20006
Phone: 800/424-8200

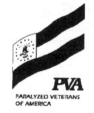

Description: Founded following World War II to bring a better life for paralyzed veterans and others with disabilities. A leader in the development of wheelchair sports in the United States. Has an active publications program. (See article on page 17.)

Sports: Instructional Training, Skiing, Wheelchair Basketball, Wheelchair Bowling, Wheelchair Tennis, Wilderness Training

Activities Offered: Tournaments; Instructional Programs; Publications; Videos

Scholarships/Awards: PVA offers the annual Jack Gerhardt Athlete-of-the-Year Award to a wheelchair athlete who "displays outstanding athletic ability and sportsmanship while contributing to the development of wheelchair sports." Named in honor of Jack Gerhardt, a native of New Jersey and a World War II paraplegic veteran, who played on one of the first wheelchair basketball teams.

Competition Events: Sponsors the U.S. Open Wheelchair Tennis Championships, the American Wheelchair Bowling Tournament, the National Wheelchair Basketball Tournament, and the National Disabled Ski Challenge. Also cosponsors the annual National Veterans Wheelchair Games with the Department of Veterans Affairs.

Workshops: Sponsors and organizes programs to enhance individual skills and to train coaches and instructors.

Manuals/Other Publications: PVA publishes two nationally recognized full-color magazines: *Sports 'n Spokes* and *Paraplegia News.*

CHAPTERS

Arizona PVA
1016 North 32nd St.
Suite 4
Phoenix, AZ 85008
Phone: 602/244-9168

Bay Area & Western PVA
3801 Miranda Ave. Bldg. 6
Palo Alto, CA 94304
Phone: 415/855-9030

Bayou PVA
3650 18th St.
Metairie, LA 41230
Phone: 504/454-1178
Toll free: 800/962-9320

Buckeye PVA
25100 Euclid Ave.
Suite 117
Euclid, OH 44117
Phone: 216/731-1017
Toll free: 800/248-2548

Cal-Diego PVA
3350 LaJolla Village Dr.
Rm 1A-118
San Diego, CA 92161
Phone: 619/450-1443

California PVA
5901 East 7th St.
Building 122 A-140
Long Beach, CA 90822
Phone: 310/494-5713

Central Florida PVA
2711 S. Design Ct.
Sanford, FL 32773
Phone: 407/328-7041 42
Toll free: 800/940-2378

Delaware-Maryland PVA
28-29 Pedders Village
Chrisiana, DE 19702
Phone: 302/368-4898
Toll free: 800/786-2039

Eastern PVA
75-20 Astoria Blvd.
Jackson Heights, NY 11370
Phone: 718/803-3782

Florida Gulf Coast PVA
121 W. 122nd Ave.
Tampa, FL 33612
Phone: 813/935-6540

Florida PVA
6200 North Andrews Ave.
Fort Lauderdale, FL 33309
Phone: 305/771-7822
Toll free: 800/683-2001

Gateway PVA
9535 Lackland Rd.
St. Louis, MO 63114
Phone: 314/427-0393

Great Plains PVA
7612 Maple St.
Omaha, NE 68134
Phone: 402/398-1422

Greater Austin Area Subchapter
Route 1 Box 117
Georgetown, TX 78626
Phone: 512/863-3043

Iowa PVA
3703 Douglas Ave.
Des Moines, IA 50310
Phone: 515/277-4782
Toll free: 800/848-0542

Kentucky-Indiana PVA
1030 Gross Ave.
Louisville, KY 40217

Phone: 502/635-6539

Lone Star PVA
3925 Forest Lane
Garland, TX 75042
Phone: 214/276-5252
Toll free: 800/583-5252

Michigan PVA
30406 Ford Rd.
Garden City, MI 48135
Phone: 313/525-5626

Mid-America PVA
5601 NW 72 St.
Suite 135
Oklahoma City, OK 73132
Phone: 405/721-7168

Mid-South PVA
VAMC 817, Rm. 2D100
1030 Jefferson Ave.
Memphis, TN 38104
Phone: 901/527-3018

Midwest Subchapter
211 Ellisonway
Independence, MO 64050
Phone: 816/461-7681

Minnesota PVA
1 Veterans Dr.
Bldg 68, Rm 217
Minneapolis, MN 55417
Phone: 612/725-2000

Mountain States PVA
1101 Syracuse St.
Denver, CO 80220
Phone: 303/322-4402
Toll free: 800/833-9400

New England PVA
1600 Providence Highway
Suite 101R
Walpole, MA 02081
Phone: 508/660-1181

North Central PVA
2204 West Madison
Sioux Falls, SD 57104
Phone: 605/336-0494

Northwest PVA
213 SW 153rd
Seattle, WA 98166
Phone: 206/241-1843

Orange Blossom Subchapter
121 West 122nd Ave.
Tampa, FL 34612
Phone: 813/935-6540

Oregon PVA
16079 SE McLoughlin Blvd.
Milwaukie, OK 97267
Phone: 503/652-0241
Toll free: 800/333-0782

Otto Smith Memorial Subchapter
403 Powhattan St.
Louisa, KY 41230
Phone: 606/638-4748

Pikes Peak Subchapter
37 Raven Hill Court
Colorado Springs, CO 80919
Phone: 719/598-0931

Pinellas Suncoast Subchapter
121 West 122nd Ave.
Tampa, FL 34612

Phone: 813/935-6540

Puerto Rico PVA
P.O. Box 363075
San Juan, PR 00936
Phone: 809/763-4471

San Antonio Subchapter
8726 Thatch
San Antonio, TX 78240
Phone: 210/647-4187

South Texas Subchapter
805 Chelsea Blvd., Suite B
Houston, TX 78240
Phone: 713/520-8782

Southeast Texas Subchapter
6911 Hearthside Drive
Sugarland, TX 77479
Phone: 713/343-9351

Southeastern PVA
4010 Deans Bridge Rd.
Hephzibah, GA 30815
Phone: 706/796-6301

Southwest Permian Basin Subchapter
Route 1, Box 357
Big Springs, TX 79720
Phone: 915/393-5304

Southwest PVA
7500 Viscount Blvd.
Suite 128
El Paso, TX 79925
Phone: 915/540-7527

Sunflower Sub-Chapter
R.R. 2 Box 58

Augusta, KS 67010
Phone: 316/775-6589

Texas PVA
805 Chelsea Blvd. Suite B
Houston, TX 77002
Phone: 713/520-8782
Toll free: 800/933-4261

Tri-State PVA
Banco Park, 1061 Main St.
North Huntingdon, PA 15642
Phone: 412/864-9323

Vaughan PVA
P.O. Box 1337
Hines, IL 60141
Phone: 708/344-8214

Virginia - Mid-Atlantic PVA
McGuire VA Medical Center

1201 Broad Rock Blvd. Bldg
507, Suite 320S
Richmond, VA 23249
Phone: 804/232-8171
Toll free: 800/852-7639

West Virginia PVA
336 Campbells Creek Dr.
Charleston, WV 25306
Phone: 304/925-9352

Wisconsin PVA
240 N. Mayfair Rd. Suite 112
Milwaukee, WI 53226
Phone: 414/475-7792
Toll free: 800/875-9782

Zia PVA
833 Gibson Blvd. SE
Albuquerque, NM 87102
Phone: 505/247-4381

Parks & Recreation Department, Santa Barbara, California

P.O. Box 1990
Santa Barbara, CA 93102-1990
Phone: 805/962-1474
Contact: Mariana de Sena

Description: Have sponsored adaptive programs for the disabled since 1979. Competitive sports program includes wheelchair tennis and wheelchair football. Also sponsor junior wheelchair sports camps for ages 5-19 in which participants are introduced to sports; coaches and trainers are disabled themselves; very non-competitive; 5-day program for about 45 kids. Those who show an interest can then join a training program for more competitive sports. Also sponsor some recreation-only "Leisure Time" programs. Sponsorship varies from program to program; individuals, civic groups, wheelchair companies, etc.

Sports: Wheelchair Football, Wheelchair Tennis, General Recreation,

Children/Youth Programs

Program/Services: "Leisure time" programs include intergenerational programs in which kids may interact with seniors through music and art. Junior wheelchair sports camps; competitive sports.

Competition Events: Annual "Blister Bowl," longest ongoing wheelchair football tournament in the United States.

Workshops: Workshops include "disability awareness days" in which able-bodied elementary school students are given an awareness of what it's like to be disabled.

Manuals/Other Publications: Bimonthly newsletter; programs for competitive sports and junior camps.

Equipment: Stock of wheelchairs and some racers

Silver Dollar Trap & Golf Club

1700 Patterson Rd
Odessa, FL 33556
Phone: 813/920-2737
Contact: Dr. Hugo or Alicia Kiem

Description: Puts on a "Chair Shoot" once a year, normally the 2nd Saturday in March. Started 6 years ago, funded through fundraising. Experienced and novice shooters are welcome. Breakfast and lunch provided. There is no membership fee.

Sports: Trap Shooting

Competition Events: Chair Shoot begins in the morning with a qualifying competition in which each participant shoots (usually 15-20 targets); after lunch, participants are put into squads: novice, intermediate, advanced, super advanced, and ladies. Trophies are given to the winners; everyone usually wins something. 50-75 participants.

How to Get Involved: Call one month in advance to register: 813/920 2737 from Nov. 1 to May 1; 914/855-5499 from May 2 to Oct. 31.

Equipment: Participants must provide their own protective eyeglasses; hearing protection, guns, and ammo is provided.

Ski for Light, Inc.

1455 West Lake Street
Minneapolis, MN 55408
Phone: 612/827-3232

Description: Ski for Light was founded in 1975. Each year Ski for Light, Inc. lays down tracks at a different winter sports area in the nation for a week of cross-country ski instruction, fitness workshops, and cultural activities. In the International Ski for Light, participants from more than a dozen countries have shared their culture, skiing skills, and experiences with Americans. In the Regional Ski for Light, regional programs are coordinated by Ski for Light "alumni" throughout the U.S., providing outdoor fitness opportunities for visually and mobility impaired persons. Both weekend and weeklong programs teach disabled individuals to cross-country ski and ice-sled.

Sports: Cross Country Skiing, Ice Sledding

Program/Services: Each disabled participant is paired with a volunteer who donates his or her skills in cross-country skiing and other fitness activities. The emphasis is on first-time participants and much time is spent on basic instruction and verbal guidance. On the ski trails guides draw word pictures of the beautiful outdoors while keeping participants on track. Mobility impaired individuals participate in the sit-ski program

Scholarships/Awards: Stipends may be available. Single rooms do not quality for stipends.

Organization Slogan: "If I can do this.../I can do anything."

Special Olympics International Headquarters

1350 New York Ave. NW
Suite 500
Washington, DC 20005-4709
Phone: 202/628-3630

TM

Description: Special Olympics is an international program of year-round sports and training and competition for children and adults with mental retardation. There are chapters established in all 50 states, the District of Columbia, Guam, the Virgin Islands, and American Samoa, and accredited programs in more than 100 countries.

Sports: Alpine Skiing, Aquatics, Athletics, Badminton, Basketball, Bowling, Cross Country Skiing, Cycling, Figure Skating, Golf, Gymnastics, Hockey, Horseback Riding, Long Distance Running, Powerlifting, Roller Skating, Soccer, Softball, Speed Skating, Table Tennis, Team Handball, Tennis, Volleyball (Standing), Walking

Program/Services: Unified Sports Program brings persons without mental retardation together on the same team with persons with mental retardation of comparable age and athletic ability. Motor Activities Training Program provides comprehensive motor activity training to individuals with severe and profound limitations.

Organization Slogan: Special Olympics Oath is "Let me win. But if I cannot win, let me be brave in the attempt."

Competition Events: Competitions are patterned after the Olympic Games. Over 15,000 Games held every year worldwide. Chapter Games held annually; National Games annually or biennially; World Games held every two years, alternating between summer and winter sports.

Workshops: Year-round training in 23 official sports

Manuals/Other Publications: Sports Skills Guide for each sport.

CHAPTERS

Alabama
560 South McDonough
Montgomery, AL 36130
Phone: 205/242-3383

Arizona
3821 East Wier Avenue
Phoenix, AZ 85040
Phone: 602/470-1080

Alaska
21-410 2nd Street
Elmendorft, AK 99506
Phone: 907/333-7006

Arkansas
1123 S. University, Suite 1017
Little Rock, AR 72204
Phone: 501/666-0423

California
501 Colorado Avenue, 2nd Fl.
Santa Monica, CA 90401
Phone: 310/451-1162

Colorado
1400 S. Colorado Blvd., Ste. 400
Denver, CO 80222
Phone: 303/691-3339

Connecticut
50 Whiting Street
Plainville, CT 06062
Phone: 203/747-5338

Delaware
Hudson Ctr.
501 Ogletown Rd. Rm. 123
Newark, DE 19711
Phone: 302/368-6818

Florida
2639 N. Monroe St. #151A
Tallahassee, FL 32303
Phone: 904/385-8178

Georgia
3772 Pleasantdale Rd.
Suite 195
Atlanta, GA 30340
Phone: 404/414-9390

Hawaii
PO 3295
Honolulu, HI 96801
Phone: 808/531-1888

Hawaii (2)
1085 S. Bretania St.
Suite 200
Honolulu, HI 96814

Idaho
8426 Fairview Avenue
Boise, ID 83704
Phone: 208/323-0482

Illinois
605 East Willow
Normal, IL 61761
Phone: 309/888-2551

Indiana
5648 West 74th Street
Indianapolis, IN 46278
Phone: 317/328-2000

Iowa
4921 Douglas
Suite 1
Des Moines, IA 50310
Phone: 515/278-2513

Kansas
5830 Woodson #106
Mission, KS 66202
Phone: 913/236-9290

Kentucky
214 W. Main Street
Frankfort, KY 40601
Phone: 502/227-7296

Louisiana
200 SW Railroad Avenue
Hammond, LA 70403
Phone: 504/345-6644

Maine
28 School Street
Gorham, ME 04038
Phone: 207/839-6030

Maryland
5020 Campbell Blvd.
Suite F
Baltimore, MD 21236
Phone: 410/931-4100

Massachusetts
PO Box 303
Hawthorne, MA 01937
Phone: 508/774-1501

Massachusetts (2)
450 Maple St.
Cottage 1
Danvers, MA 01937
Phone: 508/774-1501

Michigan
Central Michigan University
Mt. Pleasant, MI 48859
Phone: 517/774-3911

Minnesota
625 Fourth Avenue S. #1430
Minneapolis, MN 55415
Phone: 612/333-0999

Mississippi
Southern Station, Box 5174
Hattiesburg, MS 39406-5174
Phone: 601/264-7295

Missouri
1907 William Street
Jefferson City, MO 65109
Phone: 314/635-1660

Montana
3300 Third Street, NE
Great Falls, MT 59404
Phone: 406/791-2368

Nebraska
5021 S 24th St., Box 7569
Omaha, NE 68107-0569
Phone: 402/731-5007

Nevada
1101 W. Moana Lane, Suite 20
Reno, NV 89509
Phone: 702/827-2111

Nevada (2)
1700 Western Avenue Suite B
Las Vegas, NV 89102

New Hampshire
Box 311, 10 Ferry Street
Concord, MA 03301-5022
Phone: 603/226-2676

New Jersey
242 Old New Brunswick Road
Piscataway, NJ 08854
Phone: 908/562-1500

New Mexico
2403 San Mateo Blvd. NE
Suite W-10
Albuquerque, NM 87110
Phone: 505/883-5525

New York
Airport Park
3 Cornell Road
Latham, NY 12110
Phone: 518/786-8661

North Carolina
PO Box 98209
Raleigh, NC 27624-8209
Phone: 919/878-7978

North Dakota
2616 South 26th Street
Grand Forks, ND 58201
Phone: 701/746-0331

Ohio
3303 Winchester Pike
Columbus, OH 43232
Phone: 614/239-7050

Oklahoma
1860 East 15th
Tulsa, OK 74104
Phone: 918/747-9535

Oregon
3325 Yeon Avenue
Portland, OR 97210-1525
Phone: 503/248-0600

Pennsylvania
124 Washington Square
2570 Blvd. of the Generals
Norristown, PA 19403
Phone: 215/630-9450

Rhode Island
100 Jefferson Blvd.
Warwick, RI 02888
Phone: 401/463-5560

South Carolina
2615 Devine Street
Columbia, SC 29305
Phone: 803/254-7774

South Dakota
4200 South Louise Ave., #201
Sioux Falls, SD 57106
Phone: 605/361-2114

Tennessee
George Peabody College
Campus Box 39
Nashville, TN 37203
Phone: 615/322-8292

Texas
11442 North Interstate 35
Austin, TX 78753
Phone: 512/835-9873

Utah
4 Triad Center
Suite 105
Salt Lake City, UT 84180
Phone: 801/363-1111

Vermont
5 Avenue D
PO Box 1055
Williston, VT 05495
Phone: 802/863-5222

Virginia
100 W. Franklin Street
Suite 400
Richmond, VA 23220
Phone: 804/644-0071

Washington
2150 N. 107th Ave.
Suite 220
Seattle, WA 98133
Phone: 206/362-4949

Washington DC
220 Eye St NE
Suite 140
Washington, DC 20002
Phone: 202/544-7770

West Virginia
PO Box 3115
Parkersburg, WV 26103
Phone: 304/422-1868

Wisconsin
5900 Monona Dr.
Suite 301

Madison, WI 53716
Phone: 608/222-1324

Wyoming
341 East E Street #180
Casper, WY 82601
Phone: 307/235-3062

Tri Visual Services

1713 J Street
Suite 211
Sacramento, CA 95814
Phone: 916/447-7323
Contact: Elena Negrete

Description: Beep Baseball League attempting to build interest in Northern California; ages 14 to 65 may compete. Of the nine players on each team, six must be visually impaired (they are blindfolded to ensure that no one has an advantage) and three are sighted. Memberships is 25-30 with a fee of $25.00 team registration; $5.00 individual before June 1, $10 after. Affiliated with National Beep Baseball Association.

Sports: Beep Baseball

Competition Events: World Series held in August each year

Equipment: Beep baseballs and buzzing bases, built by the Telephone Pioneers of America

U.S. Fencing Association

306 Candler Street
Atlanta, GA 30307
Phone: 404/523-7421
Contact: Bill Murphy

Description: National Governing Body for Fencing in the US. Governs sport, sanctions events. The USFA Committee for the Disabled handles wheelchair fencing. Affiliated with Wheelchair Sports USA.

Sports: Fencing

U.S. Association for Blind Athletes (USABA)

33 North Institute
Colorado Springs, CO 80903
Phone: 719/630-0422
Fax: 719/630-0616

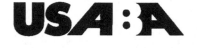

TM

Description: USABA is the official US organization to promote athletics among the legally blind. USABA is a 501(c)3 non-profit organization receiving funding from various sources including the corporate, public, and private sectors. It is a Disabled Sports Organization member of the US Olympic Committee, the International Blind Sports Association and International Paralympic Committee. It has 40 chapters. Total membership is 2,200.

Sports: Alpine Skiing, Goalball, Judo, Nordic Snow Skiing, Powerlifting, Swimming, Tandem Cycling, Wrestling

Program/Services: USABA athletes compete against both blind and sighted competition. USABA athletes—junior to elite—train at world class facilities including the Olympic Training Centers in Colorado Springs and Lake Placid, NY. Athletes range from youngsters to elite athletes competing at international events including the Paralympics. USABA also hosts developmental camps throughout the country for visually impaired children. Services include training camps and competitions.

Scholarships/Awards: Copeland Scholarship awarded to college student. Awards go to first, second, and third place finishers at National Championships. Airline Scholarships to elite athletes.

Manuals/Other Publications: *USABA Vision;* newsletter is on tape and in print

U.S. Cerebral Palsy Athletic Association (USCPAA)

3810 W. Northwest Hwy.
Suite 205
Dallas, TX 75220
Phone: 214/351-1510
Fax: 214/352-1744

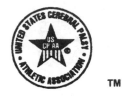

TM

Description: USCPAA is designed to provide sports training and competition opportunities for persons with cerebral palsy or who have had head injuries or strokes. Athletes may be wheelchair users or ambulatory. To insure that each athlete is competing against those with similar abilitites, the association developed an 8-part classification. This system is based on the functional level of an athlete in relation to one's sport event in a way that will allow for competition against those with similar degrees of functional ability. Since cerebral palsy manifests itself in many ways and in varying degrees, USCPAA offers a broad spectrum of sports to insure that all athletes will have the opportunity to become truly competitive. Frequently an athlete may find he or she is more competitive in one sport than in another. The Classification System is used in all individual sports, including track and field, swimming, cycling, cross country and slalom, where athletes compete only against athletes with their same classification. In the remaining sports, athletes are grouped in divisions according to classification. The only exception is powerlifting, where the division of competition is determined by body weight and gender. Athletes currently reside in over 40 states. Affiliated with DSO, USOC, and the Cerebral Palsy International Sports and Recreational Assn (CP/ISRA)

Sports: Bocci, Bowling, Cross Country Skiing, Cycling, Horseback Riding, Powerlifting, Slalom, Swimming, Team Handball, Track & Field

Competition Events: Competitions are held on the local, regional, national, and international levels.

Manuals/Other Publications: *USCPAA Update,* a newsletter

Sponsors: Sponsorship comes from the USOC, USODA, participation in the annual Combined Federal Campaign, membership dues and ongoing grant and foundation support. The goal is to raise $1,000,000 each year.

U.S. Quad Rugby Association

330 Acoma Street Apt. 607
Denver, CO 80223
Phone: 303/894-0628
Contact: Brad Mikkelsen

Description: National Governing Body for Quad Rugby in the US. Keeps constitution and bylaws, includes a governing board and executive committee; promotes the sport through clinics, sanctions national championships, regionals and sectionals. Affiliated with Wheelchair Sports USA.

Sports: Quad Rugby

Activities Offered: Put on 6 clinics a year in conjunction with PVA; locations vary by the organizations that request the clinics.

Publications: Classification manuals, referee's manuals, general quad rugby manuals; newsletter—usually 6 times a year

U.S. Rowing Association

201 S. Capital Ave.
Suite 400
Indianapolis, IN 46225
Phone: 317/237-5656

Description: Governs and promotes rowing in the US. Listed are some clubs that offer adaptive rowing programs.

Sports: Rowing

CHAPTERS

Albany Rowing Center
P.O. Box 2061
ESP Station
Albany, NY 12220-2061
Phone: 518/371-9603
Contact: Kevin Webb

American Barge Club
1321 NW 14th St., Suite 400
Miami, FL 33125
Phone: 305/325-1248
Contact: Aldo Berti

Arbor Rowing Club
P.O. Box 3128
Ann Arbor, MI 48106
Phone: 313/741-8949
Contact: Susan Prince

Bay City Rowing Club
Bay City Rowing Center
400 Lafayette
Bay City, MI 48706-5310
Phone: 517/892-5ROW
Contact: Frank Starkweather

Chelsea Rowing Club
P.O. Box 22
Norwich, CT 06360
Phone: 203/887-3511
Fax: 203/886-7649
Contact: Bob Reed

Community Rowing of Indianapolis
P.O. Box 53223
Indianapolis, IN 46253
Phone: 317/329-1960
Contact: Kris Sanford

Community Rowing, Inc.
P.O. Box 2604
Cambridge, MA 02238
Phone: 617/782-9091
Contact: Gail Sudore

Mendota Rowing Club
P.O. Box 646
Madison, WI 53701-0646
Phone: 608/233-4886
Contact: Ted Van Deburg

Moss Bay Rowing Club
135 Lake St.
Kirkland, WA 98033
Phone: 206/822-0835
Contact: Jim Clark

Northwestern State University Rowing Team
Department of Leisure Activity
and Rec. Sports
Northwestern State University
Natchitoches, LA 71497
Phone: 318/357-5921
Contact: Gene Jeffords

Philadelphia Rowing Program for the Disabled
2901 Belmont Ave.
Ardmore, PA 19003
Phone: 610/649-5463
Contact: Jonathan Hall

Rowing Unlimited
1602 South K Street
Tacoma, WA 98405
Phone: 206/591-5314
Contact: Shane Klintenstein

Toledo Rowing Club
One Maritime Plaza
Toledo, OH 43604
Phone: 313/289-3486
Contact: Jim Reisig

Upper Merion Boat Club for Competitive and Rec. Rowing
738 Hidden Valley Rd.
King of Prussia, PA 19406
Phone: 215/520-1121
Contact: Tom Pappanastasiou

U.S. Wheelchair Swimming

229 Miller St.
Middleboro, MA 02346
Phone: 508/946-1964
Contact: Joan Karpuk, Chairperson

Description: National Governing Body for Wheelchair Swimming in US. Rules for wheelchair swimming based on US Swimming organization rules, but with certain adaptations; the organization governs those adaptations. Sanctions meets and championships. Has developed a functional classification system for wheelchair swimmers so that swimmers can compete with those of similar ability. Affiliated with Wheelchair Sports USA.

Sports: Wheelchair Swimming

Program/Services: Have sponsored training camps at Olympic Training Center in Colorado Springs, and at University of California at Sacramento.

U.S. Wheelchair Weightlifting Federation/ NWAA

39 Michael Place
Levittown, PA 19057
Phone: 215/945-1964
Contact: Bill Hens

Description: The National Governing Body for Wheelchair Weightlifting, the U.S. Wheelchair Weightlifting Federation writes rules, governs the sport, and attempts to develop grassroots programs for wheelchair weightlifting. Affiliated with Wheelchair Sports USA.

Sports: Wheelchair Weight Lifting

Competition Events: Gives guidance, sanctions competitions, and governs events.

United States Blind Golfers

300 Cirondelet St.
New Orleans, LA 70130
Phone: 504/522-3203

Description: A membership organization for totally blind persons with no light perception and attested scores of 120 or less.

Sports: Golf

Veterans on the Lake

Star Route 1, Box 3420
Ely, MN 55731
Phone: 218/365-6900
Contact: Myron Tinklenberg

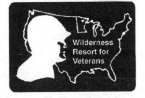

TM

Description: Private, nonprofit organization that has operated a resort for veterans since 1982; one of their main focus groups is disabled veterans. There are no special recreation programs. All groups of disabled bring their own staffs. Entire area is wheelchair accessible including Hoyer Lifts on the dock and at the pool.

Sports: Fishing, Boating, Canoeing, Shuffleboard, Tennis, Swimming, Sauna

Wheelchair Archers, USA

5318 Northport Drive
3915 Valley Road

Brooklyn Center, MN 55429
Phone: 612/533-9188
Contact: Lyn Rourke, Chairperson

Description: Formerly called American Wheelchair Archers, this association was formed to promote the sport of archery for people with disabilities. This is achieved through tournaments, publications, workshops, and programs. Membership is open to everyone involved in archery—as sport, leisure, or craft—as athlete, coach, friend, or family member. It is the only organization recognized by Wheelchair Sports, USA for purpose of selecting and training men's and women's archery teams to represent the US in the Paralympics, Pan American Games, Stoke Mandeville Tournament, and other international events. Affiliated with Wheelchair Sports USA.

Program/Services: Wheelchair Archers, USA and the National Archery Association are governed by the Federal International de Tir a 1 Arc (FITA). FITA makes and interprets all international rules and regulations for the sport. FITA rules are enforced by Wheelchair Archers, USA with the exception of a division included to provide competition for those who need to use mechanical releases, splints, and additional modified equipment. To be thoroughly versed in wheelchair archery one should be familiar with the FITA rule book available through the National Archery Association (One Olympic Plaza/Colorado Springs, CO 80909-5778).

Competition Events: Archers interested in competition primarily participate in tournaments hosted by local National Archery Association Clubs, the governing body for the sport of archery for those without disabilities. An archer using adaptive equipment will shoot in the adapted equipment division of the NWAA Archery Championship Rounds. Tournament experience is imperative when working to become a competitive archer. Local indoor and outdoor tournaments are a good place to gain experience, meet other archers, learn about equipment, and develop that competitive edge.

Tapes/Videos: Video "Archery: The Spirit is Alive." This is an informational tape covering archers who have used creativity and technology to overcome physical limitations. Contact The U.S. Archer, 7314 N. San Anna Drive, Tucson, AZ 85704. $19.95 + $2.00 shipping.

Equipment: With the aid of adaptive equipment, the quadriplegic can enjoy archery as a competitive sport or recreational activity. Certification needed to use adaptive equipment must be obtained by the archer during the medical classification to be eligible for the adaptive equipment division.

Wheelchair Athletics of the USA

30 Mayano Lane
Stamford, CT 06902
Phone: 203/967-2231
Fax: 203/327-7999
Contact: Joe Dowling

Description: National Governing Body for Track & Field in US. Governs sport, sanctions events. Affiliated with Wheelchair Sports USA.

Sports: Wheelchair Track & Field

Program/Services: Oversees Wheelchair Track & Field in the US.

Wheelchair Motorcycle Association

101 Torrey Street
Brockton, MA 02401
Phone: 508/583-8614

Description: Researches, develops, and tests types of all-terrain vehicles for use by paraplegics and quadriplegics.

Sports: Riding All-Terrain Vehicles, Motorcycling

Wheelchair Sports USA

3595 E. Fountain Blvd.
Suite L1
Colorado Springs, CO 80910
Phone: 719/574-1150

Description: Founded in 1956 as the National Wheelchair Athletic

Association, the name was changed in 1994 to Wheelchair Sports, USA. In the early years, the primary focus was organizing annual national competitions and fielding US teams. US teams have competed in world championships annually since 1960 in such countries as England, Israel, the Netherlands, Japan, Argentina, France, and other nations. Since the early 1970's additional efforts were undertaken to organize programs on more local and regional levels throughout the US. Today Wheelchair Sports USA is organized into 11 regional associations, each responsible for developing local wheelchair sports programs and for conducting qualifying meets for the National Wheelchair Games. In 1982 Wheelchair Sports USA moved to Colorado Springs to join the many other sports organizations comprising the US Olympic Committee. That association reflects a principal concern of Wheelchair Sports USA, to provide athletic experiences for the disabled athlete paralleling those of the able-bodied, from novice through elite levels. On August 11, 1984, wheelchair athletes made their formal debut in the Olympic Games with the first-ever exhibition wheelchair track events held in the Los Angeles Memorial Coliseum.

The organization has expanded its offerings to disabled youths who make up 30% of the total membership. Regional associations now conduct annual local competitions for youths aged 5-18.

From its earliest beginnings, Wheelchair Sports USA has been directed and developed by wheelchair athletes and wheelchair sports enthusiasts. By and large, the needs of the wheelchair athlete are not addressed by the vast network of athletic programs available to able-bodied persons through the educational community recreational systems. Instead, the wheelchair athlete has, with few exceptions, developed his or her own resources and opportunities, for rules and governing instruction to funding travel, equipment, and other expenses of competition. Wheelchair sports enthusiasts are involved at all levels of decision making in Wheelchair Sports USA and its constituent associations. It has remained essentially an all-volunteer organization

---

Wheelchair sports have been described as the most authentic of sports enterprises because the athletes compete and develop their own opportunities for the intrinsic values of participation and not for the promise of professional contracts or financial reward.

Sports: Archery, Fencing, Quad Rugby, Shooting (Marksmanship), Weight Lifting, Wheelchair Basketball, Wheelchair Table Tennis, Wheelchair Tennis, Wheelchair Track & Field

CHAPTERS

Appalachian Wheelchair Ath. Assn.
22 Mitchell Dr.
Abington, MD 21009
Phone: 410/669-2015 ex. 16 (W)
Fax: 410/669-7215
Contact: Gerry Herman

Dixie Wheelchair Ath. Assn.
1126 Lakeridge Ct.
Grayson, GA 30221
Phone: 404/888-0022 (W)
Fax: 404/888-9091
Contact: Linda Priest

Far West Wheelchair Ath Assn
5730 Chambertin
San Jose, CA 95118
Phone: 408/978-2828 (W)
Fax: 408/267-2834
Contact: Judy Benoit

Hawaii Wheelchair Ath Assn
P.O. Box 11120
Honolulu, HI 96828-0120
Phone: 808/943-1250 (W)
Contact: Jeff Sampaga

Michigan Wheelchair Ath Assn
14410 Vale Ct.
Sterling Hgts., MI 48312
Phone: 810/977-6123 ex. 217 (W)
Fax: 810/977-6239
Contact: Diane Winterstein

Mid-Atlantic Wheelchair Ath Assn
Box 103, WWRC

Fishersville, VA 22939
Phone: 703/332-7184 (W)
Fax: 703/332-7441
Contact: Stephen Bridge

New England Wheelchair Ath Assn
MA Hospital School
3 Randolph St.
Canton, MA 02021
Phone: 617/828-2440 ex. 388 (W)
Fax: 617/821-4086
Contact: Dick Crisafulli

North Central Wheelchair Ath Assn
Courage Center
3915 Golden Valley Rd.
Golden Valley, MN 55422
Phone: 612/520-0479 (W)
Fax: 612/520-0577
Contact: Tobe Broadrick

Northwest Wheelchair Ath Assn
3475 Winchell Ln
Billings, MT 59102
Phone: 406/259-5181 (W)
Fax: 406/259-5259
Contact: Joe Todisco

Rocky Mountain Wheelchair Ath Assn
1080 South Independence Ct.
Lakewood, CO 80226
Phone: 303/985-7525 (H)
Contact: Mary Carpenter

Southeastern Wheelchair Ath Assn
4551 Cole Rd.
Conway, SC 29526
Phone: 803/347-7486 (H)
Contact: Homer Cole

Southwest Wheelchair Ath Assn
4144 N. Central Expwy, Ste 515
Dallas, TX 45204
Phone: 214/828-1406 (SWAA Office

Contact: Paul Johnson, President

Sunshine Wheelchair Ath Assn
8301 Anglers Point Dr
Temple Terrace, FL 45204
Phone: 813/972-2000
Contact: Les Rothman

Tri-State Wheelchair Ath Assn
157-23 20th Rd
Whitesone, NY 11357
Phone: 516/296-5749
Contact: Terry Tierney

Wilderness Inquiry

1313 Fifth St. SE
Box 84
Minneapolis, MN 55414
Phone: 612/379-3858
Contact: Mr. Tracy Fredin

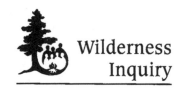

TM

Description: Nonprofit organization that sponsors wilderness activities for people of all abilities including the disabled. Offers adaptive canoe and kayak equipment.

Sports: Wilderness, Canoeing, and Kayaking

World T.E.A.M. (The Exceptional Athlete Matters) Sports

1919 South Boulevard, Suite 100
Charlotte, NC 28203
Phone: 704/344-9030
Fax: 704/344-1552
Contact: Bryan Skelton

Description: Nonprofit organization incorporated in summer of 1993, World T.E.A.M. sponsors "Challenge Events," in which physically and/or mentally disabled athletes are paired or otherwise integrated with able-bodied athletes in activities such as mountain climbing and cycling. Office in Atlanta in addition to main headquarters in Charlotte.

Activities Offered: Prior to incorporation, a World T.E.A.M. group scaled Mt. Kilimanjaro. Currently involved in AXA World Ride '95, a cycling tour around the world.

Sports: Cycling, Mountain Climbing

Programs/Services: AXA World Ride '95 is a 13,000-mile cycling tour around the world, through the US and 15 countries in Europe and Asia. There are approximately 200 athletes doing at least one of the 14 stages; about half that number are disabled. Six disabled athletes are doing all stages. Runs March 17 to November 18. Three-time Tour de France champion Greg LeMond is Honorary Chairman.

Competitions/Events: Yearly "Challenge Events"; so far have included just cycling and mountain climbing, but in the future hope to include other activities such as swimming and running.

Workshops: A 16-member cycling team (one member of which is disabled) travels around the US to train with disabled athletes in different communities.

College Opportunities

Following are profiles of the recreation and sports departments at fifteen of the premier programs in the United States, including members of the Central Intercollegiate Conference. The information provided here is based on questionnaires filled out by the program directors. While many institutions nationwide have programs for the physically challenged student as mandated by the ADA, these colleges and universities set the standard for commitment.

Ball State University

HP 222
School of Physical Education
Muncie, IN 47306-0270
Phone: 317/285-5175
Fax: 517/285-8254
Contact: Ron Davis, Associate Professor

Sports: General Recreation
Activities: Recreation, sports, intramurals
Length of Program Existence: Approx. 7 yrs.
Expansion/Cut Plans: Plans to consider interscholastic play
Governing Body: Club sports governed by Disabled Student Office & Adapted Physical Education
Tournaments/Traveling: Some travel for tournaments
Special Facilities: No separate facilities; accessible weight room, gyms, pool

Scholarships/Services: No scholarships. Tutoring and work study available.
Who should student contact? Adapted Physical Education
When should student contact? Working hours
How should student contact? By phone or mail
Number of students involved: 10-25
% Students Admitted: 100%

Strengths of Program: "Diversity; facilities; interested students to help run the programs."

Sports, Everyone!

Role of sports in life of disabled person: "Very important, the key for the future. Much needed to help build a healthy lifestyle."

Eastern Washington University

MS 66
Cheney, WA 99004-2499
Phone: 509/359-7097
Fax: 509/359-4737
Contact: Dr. Paul Green

Sports: Alpine Skiing, Cross Country Skiing
Activities: Eastern Washington University offers skiing for the disabled, using both outrigger skis and Polk sleds. The participants are mostly residents of the surrounding community, although students are welcome to join. The courses are taught by students, who receive college credit. A disabled rafting trip is also put on, once a year, generally the first Sunday in June; able-bodied students assist in this trip as well.
Special Facilities: Outrigger skis, European Polk sleds.

Scholarships/Services: No scholarships. Tutoring and work study available.
Who should student contact? Paul Green or John Cogley, 509/359-2483
Number of students involved: Approx. 200 total in skiing program; Approx. 40 in rafting

Edinboro University of Pennsylvania

Office for Students with Disabilities
Shafer Hall
Edinboro, PA 16444
Phone: 814/732-2462 voice/tdd
Fax: 814/732-2866
Contact: Dr. Robert McConnell, Ass't Dir., Office for Students with Disabilities

Sports: Air Rifle, Archery, Basketball, Football, Quad Rugby, Road Racing, Scuba Diving, Swimming, Table Tennis, Track & Field, Weight Lifting
Length of Program Existence: Approx. 17 yrs.
Expansion/Cut Plans: Maintain current levels

Governing Body: WAA, NWBA, LASA, USCPAA
Tournaments/Traveling: Teams travel to tournaments
Special Facilities: Separate weight room, exercise room, plans for expanded facility

Scholarships/Services: Tutoring and work study available.
Who should student contact? Contact the Office for Students with Disabilities for further information.
Number of students involved: Approx. 50

Strengths of Program: "Support services for students: transportation, wheelchair maintenance, attendant care, adaptive computers, occupational therapy services."
Notes: Charlotte W. Newcombe Foundation awards the University $15,000 to $22,000 a year for special disability expenses, scholarships, internships, and partial tuition. The OSD provides special services for students with learning disabilities. The Nursing Station allows close monitoring of health concerns related to a disability. The Life Skills Center offers training to disabled students to help them with both personal independence and academics. The Pennsylvania Office for Vocational Rehabilitation offers support to the OSD and provides special equipment and educational programs at Edinboro. The Bureau of Blindness and Visual Services in Pennsylvania and Edinboro University offers an orientation program to visually impaired students

Gallaudet University

800 Florida Ave. NE
Washington, DC 20002
Phone: 202/651-5603
Fax: 202/651-5274

Sports: Baseball, Basketball, Cross Country, Football, Soccer, Tennis, Track & Field, Volleyball (Standing), Wrestling
Length of Program Existence: 112 yrs.
Expansion/Cut Plans: Maintain current level.
Governing Body: NCAA; governing body for football is athletic department and university
Intramural/Interscholastic: Starting in '95-'96 season, football will be independent and team will play more clubs
Conferences: NCAA Div. III: Capital Athletic Conference, Mason-Dixon Conference
Tournaments/Traveling: All sports involve tournaments and travel

Special Facilities: All buildings on campus have TTY's. Also, fire alarms are loud and vibrating with strobe lights. Close captioned TV also available.

Scholarships/Services: There is some vocational rehab aid available from state and federal sources, but it is not talent-based. Tutoring and work study available.
Who should student contact? Joe Fritsch, Athletic Director
Conferences: NCAA Div. III: Capital Athletic Conference, Mason-Dixon Conference

Strengths of Program: "Offer opportunities that other colleges offer, but for people who have a hearing loss. Can offer hearing impaired students more because of communication. Other students who come from a similar background. Located in Washington DC."
Advice: "Study hard; academics must be a priority."
Role of sports in life of disabled person: "Important to a deaf person as to anyone else. Important part of life for physical fitness, but also an important part of school life; adds balance to a person's life. Also important for self-discipline, self-motivation, time-management, and teamwork."
Notes: Entire undergraduate population is hearing impaired. School was founded in 1864; Abraham Lincoln signed the charter. A few of the athletic teams (men's and women's basketball, for example) have cuts; most do not. Teams tend to grow and shrink in relation to the World Games for the Deaf (which occur every four years): a year or two before the Games, teams tend to grow, as athletes may be competing in order to train for the Games; a year or two after, teams tend to shrink. While Gallaudet has no direct involvement with the Games, many of its athletes compete in them. The next World Games for the Deaf will be in 1997. *See* American Athletic Association for the Deaf (AAAD) in the "Associations" section for more information on the World Games.

Idaho State University

Cooperative Wilderness Handicapped Outdoor Group
Box 8118, Pond Student Union
Pocatello, ID 83209
Phone: 208/236-3912
Contact: Jeff Brandt

Activities: Wilderness activities/trips; classes in adaptive swimming, water skiing, snow skiing, weight training, and aerobics may be taken for credit through the Physical Education Department of Idaho State University. Trips include, but are not limited to, whitewater rafting, rock climbing, sky diving, hiking, camping, fishing, kayaking, sailing, pheasant hunting, dog sledding, and riding all-terrain vehicles.

Length of Program Existence: 14 yrs.
Governing Body: Elected board of directors.
Intramural/Interscholastic: More of a regional self-help group than a college-run University activity.
Tournaments/Traveling: Travel.
Special Facilities: Adaptive snow and water skiing equipment.

Scholarships/Services: There is a fund used to defray cost of trips for those with financial need. Tutoring and work study available.
Who should student contact? Jeff Brandt
When should student contact? Anytime
How should student contact? Phone call or letter
% Students Admitted: 100%

Strengths of Program: "From within the security of a supportive peer group, individuals are encouraged to challenge their limits and expand their horizons. Activities are directed by group consensus and are not watered down or contrived. Through self-direction, participants gain the skills to initiate activities independently or for the benefit of the group....Active participants determine what activities they wish to plan."

San Jose State University

Department of Human Performance
College of Applied Sciences and Arts
San Jose, CA 95192-0054
Phone: 408/924-3010
Fax: 408/924-3053
Contact: Dr. Nancy Megginson, Coordinator of Adapted Physical Activity, Undergraduate/Graduate Program

Activities: The SJSU Department of Human Performance Adapted Physical Activity program has been co-sponsor of various disability sport training and competition at the local, regional, and national levels. In the last five years, it has supported the following events: 1992 U.S. Quad Rugby Association National Championships; 1992 National Wheelchair Basketball/Paralyzed Veterans of America National Training Camp; 1994 National Wheelchair Basketball Association National Tournament; 1994 Paralympic Wheelchair Basketball Training Camp. 1990 - current: Various local and sectional wheelchair basketball tournaments; various local and sectional quad rugby tournaments; annual WSUSA (Wheelchair Sports USA) Far West region developmental sports camp for youth who use wheelchairs; 1995 DS/USA (Disabled Sports USA) Adapted Physical Fitness Leadership training site. In addition to the listed events, SJSU Department of Human Performance Adapted Physical Activity Program has, also, supported various developmental sports camps and training programs for individuals who have blindness or mental retardation in cooperation with the USABA and Special Olympics, respectively. In 1992, a SJSU student aquatic club called Diving with Disabilities (DWD) was established through the SJSU Adapted Physical Activity Program. DWD's primary purpose is to improve the quality of life for students with physical disabilities by providing specialized training in snorkeling and scuba. The club meets once a week for a two and one-half hour period, utilizing the SJSU indoor pool. Aquatic activities include snorkeling, scuba, and kayak experiences. Individuals with disabilities are paired with non-disabled student volunteers from SJSU adapted physical education classes. Over 40 individuals with disabilities and their non-disabled "buddies" have participated in some aspect of DWD's weekly training program.

Length of Program Existence: 5 yrs.

Expansion/Cut Plans: Expansion plans focus on development of an adapted physical activity facility called "Speed City Sports Center." Will include offices, classrooms, library, conference space, locker rooms, gymnasium, weight training/cardiovascular equipment, exercise physiology, biomechanic/stress management/motor control laboratories, athletic training room, and track/field area. "Speed City Sports Center" will be the first in the nation to offer disability sport organizations, in cooperation with SJSU, a fully adapted facility which meets and exceeds the requirements of sanctioned local, regional, national, and international competition. It also will provide both the public and private sector an opportunity to learn, explore, and understand the individual with a disability.

Special Facilities: San Jose State University is California's oldest public institution of higher education. SJSU stresses excellence in both classroom instruction and "hands-on" experience. Many of the university's 2000 full and part-time faculty are active in scholarly, laboratory, and field research, providing increased opportunities for students, as co-workers, to gain valuable practical education. The Human Performance Department at SJSU is a multifaceted department within the College of Applied Arts and Sciences. Four basic academic programs reflect the department's involvement within the university: General Education; Physical Education Activity; Undergraduate; and Graduate. Within the department, there are 8000 general education and physical education activity students, 350 undergraduate majors, and 80 graduate students. There are also 25 full-time and 38 part-time faculty who teach in the department. The facilities within the Department of Human Performance offer fully equipped laboratories in exercise physiology, biomechanics, athletic training, and motor behavior. These labs contain the state-of-the-art equipment as well as an array of computer systems and related software. High speed filming, video equipment, including an underwater setup, and audio-visual production are available. Physical facilities include laboratories, classrooms, several gymnasia, two aquatic areas, outdoor fields, and court areas.

Scholarships/Services: Various academic awards/scholarships (up to $500) are available at the college and university levels. In addition, the SJSU Disabled Student Services holds an annual awards ceremony, honoring an outstanding student with disability. Tutoring and work study available.

Notes: The goal of the SJSU undergraduate adapted physical activity training program is to provide the student with the necessary skills and knowledge to work with persons with disabilities in a physical activity framework. The student will learn, through didactic course work, extensive practicum opportunities, and personal research, the necessary components required to pursue a career in adapted physical activity. Types of available employment opportunities for persons with a degree in adapted physical activity include working in private schools, health clubs, corporate fitness centers, recreational settings, hospitals, rehabilitation centers, infant and early childhood programs, senior centers, and disability sports organizations. For students who wish to pursue a teaching credential in adapted physical education, employment in public schools is an additional option. Graduate adapted physical activity professional preparation is intended to increase the breadth and depth of knowledge/competence of the student currently providing services in the field to individuals with disabilities. Practical research application and enhanced professional involvement is encouraged at this level.

Southern Illinois University at Carbondale

Lingle Hall
Room 118
Carbondale, IL 62901-4710
Phone: 618/453-2121
Fax: 618/453-5152
Contact: Kim Martin, Wheelchair Basketball Coach

Sports: Quad Rugby, Wheelchair Basketball, Wheelchair Racquetball, Wheelchair Tennis, Wheelchair Track, Fitness (disabled students are matched with fitness partners), Weight Training, Swimming, Aerobics, Range of Motion/Stretching, Bowling, Outdoor Activities (e.g., fishing, rappelling, rock climbing, water skiing).
Length of Program Existence: Approx. 20 yrs.
Expansion/Cut Plans: No plans to cut; expansion is always a struggle.
Governing Body: Not officially sanctioned by NCAA, although wheelchair basketball does operate under the rules of the NCAA. Office of Student Affairs governs program.
Intramural/Interscholastic: Wheelchair basketball is interscholastic; wheelchair tennis is considered extramural, but for all practical purposes functions as an intramural sport.
Conferences: Central Intercollegiate Conference
Special Facilities: Student rec center is totally accessible to disabled. There is some special adaptive equipment, e.g., adaptive weight training equipment and wheelchair basketball, tennis, and track chairs.

Scholarships/Services: No scholarships at present; however, there is $4600 allocated for tuition waiver money, which is used as a recruiting tool. Tutoring and work study available.
Selection Criteria: Based on academics, financial need, and whether student will be a good role model.
Who makes decision? Kim Martin makes the selection and VP of Student Affairs makes final decision
Who should student contact? Kim Martin or Kathy Hollister
How should student contact? Phone call is easiest.
Number of students involved: 80
% Students Admitted: 100%
Avg SAT Score: 750
Avg ACT Score: 18-21
Avg GPA: 2.5

Strengths of Program: "In other schools, the primary focus is competition; SIU offers competitive and recreational opportunities so that a wider range of students can get involved."

Advice: "Make academics your first consideration. A lot of kids may want to attend SIU simply because it has wheelchair athletics, but this should not be the only or most important factor in the decision."

Role of sports in life of disabled person: Kim Martin, who is paraplegic, speaks from personal experience when she says "Sports can play a huge role as a type of motivator for goal-setting, self-esteem, academics, and socialization."

Southwest State University

1501 State Street
Marshall, MN 56258-1598
Phone: 507/537-7271
Fax: 507/537-6578
Contact: Lew Shaver, Wheelchair Basketball Coach (retired)
Other contact: Bob Johnson

Sports: Wheelchair Basketball
Activities: All phys. ed. classes are open and disabled student population is mainstreamed in this regard.
Length of Program Existence: 26 yrs.
Expansion/Cut Plans: Always looking to expand.
Governing Body: Athletic department.
Intramural/Interscholastic: Program is intercollegiate.
Conferences: NCAA Div. II, Central Intercollegiate Conference
Tournaments/Traveling: Yes
Special Facilities: Some sport chairs are provided; most students provide their own. No other special facilities; program's philosophy is that disabled students should not be separated from the rest of the student population.

Scholarships/Services: Yes. A specific amount is available to an unspecified number of athletes. Tutoring and work study available.
Scholarship Selection Criteria: NCAA guidelines: Academics and talent
Who makes decision? Lew Shaver makes recommendation, Athletic Director makes final decision.
Who should student contact? Lew Shaver
How should student contact? Phone call or mail.
Number of students involved: 10-14

% Students Admitted: Majority.

Strengths of Program: "Legitimacy—the program is a part of the athletics program and not part of disabled student services."

Advice: "Students should be responsible for getting as much information as they can about wheelchair basketball, and also should be responsible for giving themselves as many options as possible."

Role of sports in life of disabled person: "The role of sports in the life of a disabled person should be the same as it is in anyone else's life. It is identical if you allow it to be."

Temple University

1858 N. Broad Street 108-00
Philadelphia, PA 19121
Phone: 215/204-1267; TTY 204-1786
Fax: 215/204-3800
Contact: Steve Young, Director—Recreation Services
Other contact: Tribit Green, Rec Specialist (Adapted Rec)

Sports: Wheelchair Basketball, General Recreation
Activities: Specialized assistance provided for additional activities. Activities include but are not limited to: swimming, physical conditioning, rowing, horseback riding, road racing, bowling, and wheelchair sports.
Length of Program Existence: 8 yrs.
Expansion/Cut Plans: No plans for expansion. Cuts are always possible due to budget constraints, yet no immediate plans.
Governing Body: Wheelchair basketball is part of the NWBA; they have had membership in the C.I.C. at times depending on finances and roster.
Intramural/Interscholastic: Wheelchair basketball is extramural, similar to a club where they play other clubs. They do travel regionally.
Special Facilities: Facilities utilized are the same as utilized for the able-bodied population. No separate facilities.

Scholarships/Services: No scholarships. Tutoring and work study available.
Who should student contact? Tribit Green
When should student contact? Weekdays 8:30-4:30
How should student contact? Letter or phone contact is best.
Number of students involved: Approx. 29
% Students Admitted: 100%

Strengths of Program: "Varied opportunities for students with disabilities. Staff member that helps to coordinate, advocate and program for these individuals. Competitive wheelchair program."

Advice: "Make sure they are choosing an institution based on academics as the priority, extracurricular activities as a secondary concern."

Role of sports in life of disabled person: "Because physical activity and social health both play an important role in college life, Recreation Services offers extracurricular opportunities for physically disabled students. The goals of the adapted Recreation program are: 1) to introduce students to lifelong leisure skills; 2) promote total participation in college life."

Notes: Recreational activities are coordinated by a Certified Therapeutic Recreation Specialist (CRTS). Goals of the Adapted Rec program are: 1) to introduce students to various life-long leisure skills; 2) to identify and utilize accessible leisure and recreation facilities in the community that will be available after college; and 3) to promote total participation in college life.

The Ohio State University

337 W. 27th Ave
Rm. 106
Columbus, OH 43210
Phone: 614/292-7671
Fax: 614/292-4105

Sports: General Recreation
Activities: Aquatic and conditioning programs. Also other sports activities including wheelchair basketball, football, golf, T-ball, softball, quad rugby, badminton, swimming, volleyball, racquetball, track & field, weightlifting, table tennis, and tennis. All activities are intramural. Also individual recreation and outdoor pursuits including archery, chess, self-defense, yoga, bicycling, camping, canoeing, and downhill and cross country skiing.
Length of Program Existence: 11 yrs.
Expansion/Cut Plans: No to cuts, possibly to expand.
Governing Body: University
Intramural/Interscholastic: ARISE (Adapted Recreation and Intramural Sport Enrichment) Program (formerly Project Leisure Education Participation) is a university leisure/recreation program for individuals with physical and/or sensory disabilities, designed to serve ages 6 months through adult, students and non-students in the Central Ohio

111

Community. Staffed by students who are regular or Federal Work Study Employees, volunteers, Field Experience or Community Service individuals.

Special Facilities: Modified Universal machine for participants. Pools have attached lifts.

Scholarships/Services: No scholarships right now. Tutoring and work study available.

Who should student contact? Jayne Allison

When should student contact? Afternoons

How should student contact? Telephone or e-mail.

Number of students involved: 20 students, 80 community members

% Students Admitted: 100%

Strengths of Program: "We provide a place for participants to fulfill their physical/social needs."

Advice: "Be active."

Role of sports in life of disabled person: "It helps to improve the quality of their lives."

University of Arizona

1540 E. Second St.
Tucson, AZ 85721
Phone: 502/621-5178
Fax: 502/621-9423
Contact: David Herr-Cardillo, Director of Wheelchair Athletic Programs

Sports: Quad Rugby, Skiing, Strength and Conditioning Programs, Wheelchair Basketball, Wheelchair Tennis, Wheelchair Track

Activities: Wheelchair basketball is offered on 2 levels: Competitive—October to March. Wildchairs team is a member of the National Wheelchair Basketball Association. Recreational—The off-season is from April to September. A good time to learn the sport. Limited instruction is available.

Length of Program Existence: 21 yrs.

Expansion/Cut Plans: Expansion depends on funding. No plans to cut.

Governing Body: Sanctioned by NWBA, USORA, Wheelchair Sports, USA

Intramural/Interscholastic: Activities are designed as club sport status.

Tournaments/Traveling: Tournament and seasonal play do occur.

Special Facilities: First-rate athletic and recreational facilities. Some separate facilities exist but most are integrated.

Scholarships/Services: Scholarships available. Tutoring and work study available.
Scholarship Selection Criteria: Athletic ability.
Who makes decision? Dave Herr-Cardillo
Who should student contact? Dave Herr-Cardillo
When should student contact? 1 pm to 5 pm Mountain Time
How should student contact? Phone call—502/621-5178
Number of students involved: 60

Strengths of Program: "Beautiful climate of the Southwest; the chance to compete athletically in an established sports program."
Role of sports in life of disabled person: "Essential. In today's society, athletics/recreation are a part of everyone's life."

University of Illinois

Div. of Rehabilitation Education Services
1207 S. Oak Street
Champaign, IL 61820
Phone: 217/333-1970 or 333-4603
Contact: Brad Hedrick
Other contact: Marty Morse

Sports: Quad Rugby, Wheelchair Basketball—Men's, Wheelchair Basketball—Women's, Wheelchair Track/Road Racing
Activities: There are other recreation opportunities for the disabled in addition to the competitive sports; contact school for details.
Length of Program Existence: 47 yrs.
Expansion/Cut Plans: No plans to cut; expansion depends on resources
Governing Body: Wheelchair Sports USA: Basketball, National Wheelchair Basketball Association; Quad Rugby: US Quad Rugby Association
Intramural/Interscholastic: Only Men's Basketball is technically interscholastic; however, Womens' Basketball, Track & Field, and Quad Rugby have all the training and coaching resources of traditional interscholastic models, even though they don't compete interscholastically.
Conferences: Central Intercollegiate Conference
Tournaments/Traveling: Yes, for Men's Basketball

Sports, Everyone!

Special Facilities: All special equipment required is provided; however due to budget constraints, costs of supplies, e.g., tires, are often the student's responsibly.

Scholarships/Services: The Division of Rehabilitation Education Services has a scholarship endowment. Tuition waivers, which cover the differential between in-state and out-of-state tuition, are offered to 7 students in Men's & Women's Wheelchair Basketball. Tutoring and work study available.

Selection Criteria: Depends on rosters and in which sports athletes are needed; student's sports history, performance, potential. Because of the University's scholastic requirements for entry, academics are assumed.

Who makes decision? Brad Hedrick

Who should student contact? Brad Hedrick

When should student contact? A year in advance of entry

How should student contact? Phone or letter; videotape is often requested after initial contact

Number of students involved: 45

% Students Admitted: At 45 students currently, program is not at a point where they need to reject any students; if the situation should arise in the future, intramural or club programs could be created to accommodate the overflow students.

Conferences: Central Intercollegiate Conference

Strengths of Program: Brad Hedrick: "The University of Illinois is consistently ranked among the finest institutions in the United States. The breadth of the wheelchair athletics programs, the coaching expertise, and training opportunities are also great strengths." From Media Guide: The University of Illinois Division of Rehabilitation Education Services is recognized as a world leader in the education of persons with disabilities as well as research training and programming in rehabilitation. It pioneered the development of architectural design standards which served as benchmarks for accessibility standards nationally and internationally. Members of the coaching staff are recognized as among the best in the world; coaches have won tournament championships; have themselves participated or coached participants, record holders, and medalists in the Boston Marathon, the Pan American Games, the Paralympics, and the Olympics, including 5-time Boston Marathon World Record holder and Olympic Silver Medalist Jean Driscoll and National Wheelchair Basketball Hall of Famer and Olympic Gold Medalist Sharon Hedrick.

Advice: "Foremost criteria is performance in the classroom. The ability to set and attain goals is as important in the classroom as it is in athletics for students to perform to their potential; the ultimate goal of the

program is to help students perform to their potential."
Role of sports in life of disabled person: "We all seek and desire challenge in life; sports is one means to find challenge. Sports affords a unique opportunity to fill a void in the self-concept of a person with disabilities. It helps to socialize athletes with disabilities as well as helping them to avoid negative lifestyle behaviors."

Notes: The rehabilitation service fraternity, Delta Sigma Omicron, sponsors numerous service projects.

University of Nebraska at Lincoln

103 S. Stadium
Lincoln, NE 68588
Phone: 402/472-3644
Fax: 402/472-2005
Contact: Leah Hall Dorothy, Assistant Director for Sport Clubs and Special Programs, Office of Campus Recreation

Sports: Wheelchair Basketball, Wheelchair Racquetball, Wheelchair Tennis
Length of Program Existence: 2 yrs.
Expansion/Cut Plans: No plans to cut; expansion depends on student interest
Governing Body: Office of Campus Recreation
Intramural/Interscholastic: Basketball is interscholastic; tennis and racquetball are intraclub
Special Facilities: Facilities are not separate, but they are accessible. 8300 sq. foot weight room, racquetball courts, 30 tennis courts, 8 all-purpose courts; accessible pool and indoor football field. Sports chairs are available.

Scholarships/Services: No scholarships. Tutoring and work study available.
Who should student contact? Leah Hall Dorothy, 55 Campus Recreation Ctr, 68588-0232
Number of students involved: 25-30
% Students Admitted: 100%

Strengths of Program: "Young program just getting started—lots of flexibility. Program is under student services umbrella, so lots of help is available to disabled students."
Advice: "We welcome students of all abilities. Include sports in your

college life for health and to be a well-rounded student."
Role of sports in life of disabled person: "To be mentally active and well-rounded, fitness and sports is important. Students can find a lifetime activity that they will enjoy."

University of Texas at Arlington

PO Box 19079
Arlington, TX 76019
Phone: 817/273-3364; TDD 817/273-3323
Fax: 817/794-5037
Contact: Jim Hayes, Director of Office for Students with Disabilities

Sports: Wheelchair Basketball
Activities: The Office for Students with Disabilities offers an array of services for disabled students including pre-registration; personal, academic, and career counseling; wheelchair repair; adaptive testing; note copying; adaptive exercise and sports activities (EXSA) courses; wheelchair athletics; and agency interface. The director encourages all disabled students to visit the office prior to registration to receive information on a variety of services designed for specific disabilities.
Length of Program Existence: 6 yrs.
Expansion/Cut Plans: As funds permit; the next scholarshipped sport will be Intercollegiate Tennis
Governing Body: National Wheelchair Basketball Association
Conferences: Central Intercollegiate Conference
Tournaments/Traveling: Yes
Special Facilities: All facilities are accessible. Wheelchair basketball locker doors and wheelchair repair are separate.

Scholarships/Services: Currently offer 7 full scholarships in basketball. Tutoring and work study available.
Scholarship Selection Criteria: Previous sports activity; Degree specific
Who makes decision? Head Coach Jim Hayes
Who should student contact? Jim Hayes
When should student contact? January for following September
How should student contact? Letter of Interest
Number of students involved: 15
% Students Admitted: 5%
Avg SAT Score: 1000

Strengths of Program: "We treat the wheelchair athlete as we do all

athletes. Academics first, sports second."
Advice: "Choose your institution based on academic objectives."
Role of sports in life of disabled person: "Essential to well-rounded health and physical demands of living."

University of Wisconsin at Whitewater

Wheelchair Athletics & Recreation Office
Williams Center, U-W Whitewater
Whitewater, WI 53190
Phone: 414/472-3169
Fax: 414/472-5210
Contact: Michael Frogley, Coordinator of Wheelchair Athletics and Recreation; Mike Lenser, Physical Therapist 414/472-1524; Jim Truesdale, Disabled Student Services, 414/472-4711

Sports: Hang Gliding, Horseback Riding, Swimming, Wheelchair Basketball, Wheelchair Football, Wheelchair Track
Activities: Wheelchair Basketball and Swimming are competitive. The other sports are recreational. There is also an extensive junior program in all of these areas. In addition there are exercise and physical therapy programs available. Membership includes 80 university students and 80 juniors.
Length of Program Existence: Since 1973
Expansion/Cut Plans: Plan is to expand the program competitively and add wheelchair track and quad rugby
Governing Body: NCAA governs the competitive sports while recreational sports are governed by NWBA and NWAA.
Intramural/Interscholastic: Competitive sports are interscholastic and involve extensive tournament play. Intramurals are wheelchair football and basketball and involve tournaments and travel.
Conferences: NCAA; NWBA; NWAA
Tournaments/Traveling: Yes
Special Facilities: All facilities and equipment are adapted for use by individuals with a disability.

Scholarships/Services: A small number of scholarships are offered along with a limited number of out-of-state tuition waivers. Tutoring and work study available.
Who makes decision? Determined by scholarship committee and University Admissions
Who should student contact? Contact Michael Frogley or John Truesdale

When should student contact? As soon as the student is interested for contact.

How should student contact? Either by phone or in writing.

Number of students involved: 160

% students admitted: All who meet admission requirements, plus some exceptions are recommended.

Conferences: NCAA; NWBA; NWAA

Avg ACT Score: 21

Avg GPA: 2.75

Strengths of Program: "Provides diverse opportunities along with an opportunity for individuals to develop their own areas of interest. On the cutting edge of program and athletic developments for individuals with a disability. Also has an extensive Junior program which holds exciting and challenging summer camps in such areas as Wheelchair Basketball, Wheelchair Sports and Ultimate Adventure. The Ultimate Adventure camp will include specialized athletics including a challenge course, rock climbing, rapelling, white-water rafting, camping, hang gliding and water skiing. The wheelchair sports camp introduces youths to basketball, tennis, fitness, training, swimming, martial arts and water skiing. Participants to camps are ages 8-18 who have a mobility impairment as their primary disability. All levels of mobility are encouraged to attend. Financial aid for the camp usually takes the form of local service clubs and special education sources in your school district."

Advice: "Apply early to allow for planning; show initiative by following up with phone calls; plan a campus visit."

Role of sports in life of disabled person: "It is a unique area that allows for the development of the total person through the use of physical activity and athletics to develop the total person."

Notes: University holds summer camps for pre-college students: Junior Warhawk Wheelchair Basketball Camp, Warhawk Ultimate Adventure Camp, and the Junior Warhawk Wheelchair Sports Camp. The Junior Warhawk Outreach Program is provided throughout the school year and trains young athletes in competitive track and basketball. Direct questions to Michael Frogley, Sheila Williams, Vicky Coons, or Anje Olander.

Wright State University

Intramural and Recreational Sports
E009 Student Union
Dayton, OH 45435
Phone: 513/873-5815
Fax: 513/873-5527

Sports: Aquatics, Biking, Bowling, Quad Rugby, Wheelchair Basketball, Wheelchair Football, Wheelchair Softball, Wheelchair Tennis, Wheelchair Track

Activities: Wright State is a leader in providing support services and an accessible campus for students with physical and learning disabilities. The Office of Disability Services offers physical and academic support services for students with disabilities. Physical support services include attendant care, campus mobility orientation for visually impaired students, and other services to promote independence. Academic support services include test proctoring, taped textbooks, and other academic aids. Students are urged to contact Disability Services before enrolling to plan for necessary support services. The Office of Disability Services also helps students with disabilities plan and implement career choices. A broad range of adapted athletic, intramural, and recreational activities are also available to students with disabilities. Sports are divided into intramurals and clubs. Intramural sports are 1) wheelchair basketball; 2) wheelchair football; 3) wheelchair tennis; 4) wheelchair softball; 5) adapted aquatics; 6) bowling. Club sports include 1) women's wheelchair basketball; 2) men's wheelchair basketball; 3) wheelchair tennis; 4) wheelchair track; 5) quad rugby; 6) biking.

Length of Program Existence: 24 yrs.

Expansion/Cut Plans: Plans to expand.

Governing Body: Club sports: National Governing Body of each particular disabled sport.

Tournaments/Traveling: Yes

Special Facilities: No special facilities; students have use of University facilities at Student Union and Nutter Center.

Scholarships/Services: Scholarships available. Tutoring and work study available.

Scholarship Selection Criteria: GPA, leadership, contribution

Who makes decision? Selection committees

Who should student contact? Admissions, E148 Student Union, 513/873-5700

Number of students involved: Approx. 200

Strengths of Program: "Opportunities for individual involvement, leadership, and participation with a diverse campus community sensitive to student development."

Advice: "Make a campus visit—contact Campus Orientation, W034 Student Union, 513/873-5570."

Role of sports in life of disabled person: "An excellent opportunity to learn about yourself, others, and life."

Camps

This information is supplied by the American Camping Association which accredits all kinds of camps across the country. For further information which the ACA can provide, please call toll free 1-800-428-CAMP.

ALABAMA

ASCCA

PO Box 21
Jackson Gap, AL 36861
Phone: 205/825-9226
Resident Camp
Director: Jerry Bynum
Operator: Alabama Easter Seal Society, Camp ASCCA. PO Box 21, Jackson Gap, AL 36861 205/825-9226
Clientele/Fees: Coed from 2 to 99, 6 days for $365.00, 11 days for $560.00
Operating Season: 10/01 to 9/30
Capacity: 220
Facilities: Cabins, Lodge, Tents
Camp's Comments: Camperships available for need, Alabama disabled camper only.
General Physical Disabilities, Hearing Impairment, Visual Impairments

ARKANSAS

Camp Aldersgate, Inc.

2000 Aldersgate Road
Little Rock, AR 72205
Phone: 501/225-1444
Resident Camp

Sports, Everyone!

Director: Sarah M. Spencer
Operator: Women's Div/Board of Global Ministries, UMC, 2000 Aldersgate Rd., Little Rock, AR 72205 501/225-1444
Clientele/Fees: Coed from 6 to 16, 5 days for $325.00
Operating Season: 1/1 to 12/31
Capacity: 45
Facilities: Cabins
Camp's Comments: Trad. camp for children & youth w/medical and physical disability.
Hearing Impairment, Mobility Limitations

CALIFORNIA

Bloomfield

35375 Mulholland Hgwy.
Malibu, CA 90265
Phone: 310/457-5330
Resident Camp
Director: Lisa Torres
Operator: Diabetic Youth Foundation, 1954 Mt Diablo Blvd Ste. A, Walnut Creek, CA 94596 510/937-3393
Clientele/Fees: Coed from 6 to 22, Adults from 21 +
Operating Season: 6/21 to 8/21
Capacity: 220
Facilities: Cabins
Camp's Comments: Camp serves blind & visually impaired children and families
Visual Impairments

Camp Krem

102 Brook Lane
Boulder Creek, CA 91723
Phone: 408/338-3210
Resident Camp
Director: Michael Gaboury
Operator: Camping Unlimited for Retarded Children Inc., 1302 Albina Avenue, Berkeley, CA 94706 415/527-4488
Clientele/Fees: Coed from 4 to 70, 12 days for $660.00

Operating Season: 6/14 to 8/22
Facilities: Cabins, Lodges, Tents
Camp's Comments: Camp serves people of all ages and all handicaps
General Physical Disabilities, Mobility Limitations

Camp-A-Lot

1550 Hotel Circle North #400
San Diego, CA 92108-2910
Phone: 619/574-7575
Resident Camp
Director: Jaculin "Lin" Taylor
Operator: Association for Retarded Citizens—San Diego, CA 92108-2910, 619/574-7575
Clientele/Fees: Coed from 7 to 18, adults from 13 to 80, 5 days for $285.00, 7 days for $399.00, 8 days for $456.00, 10 days for $570
Operating Season: 6/28 to 8/22
Capacity: 100
Facilities: Cabins, Dorms, Lodge, Tent
Camp's Comments: Resident camp for developmentally disabled children & adults
Mobility Limitations

Costanoan

13851 Stevens Canyon Rd.
Cupertino, CA 95014
Phone: 408/867-1115
Resident Camp
Director: Debbie Blue
Operator: Crippled Children's Soc of Santa Clara County, 2851 Park Ave., Santa Clara, CA 95050, 408/243-7861
Clientele/Fees: Coed from 5 to 18, Adults from 18 to 90, Adults from 55 to 90, 2 days for $98.82, 8 days for $398.00
Operating Season: 1/1 to 12/31
Capacity: 100
Facilities: Lodge
Camp's Comments: Serve a wide range of disabilities. Year-round respite.
General Physical Disabilities, Mobility Limitations

Easter Seal Camp Harmon

16403 Highway 9
Boulder Creek, CA 95006
Phone: 408/338-3383
Resident Camp
Director: Jane Carr
Operator: Easter Seal Society, 9010 Soquel Drive Ste 1, Aptos, CA 95003-4002, 408/684-2166
Clientele/Fees: Coed from 8 to 60, 6 days for $534.00, 12 days for $1068.00, 3 days for $168.00
Operating Season: 1/1 to 12/31
Capacity: 150
Facilities: Cabins, Lodge
Camp's Comments: Barrier free, able to serve severely disabled campers.
General Physical Disabilities, Mobility Limitations

Joan Mier

11677 E. Pacific Coast Hwy
Malibu, CA 90265
Phone: 213/874-3300
Resident Camp
Director: Lee Ann Gabler
Operator: Crippled Children's Society, 11677 E. Pacific Coast Hwy, Malibu, CA 90265, 213/874-3300
Clientele/Fees: Coed from 7 to 65, 7 days for $630.00, 8 days for $720.00
Operating Season: 6/18 to 8/24
Capacity: 100
Facilities: Cabins
Camp's Comments: All facilities are wheelchair accessible.
General Physical Disabilities, Mobility Limitations

Enchanted Hills Camp

34110 Mt Veeder Rd.
Napa, CA 94558
Phone: 707/224-4023

Resident Camp
Director: Theresa Duncan
Operator: Lighthouse for the Blind
Clientele/Fees: Coed from 8 to 18, Adults from 35 to 99, 5 days for $300.00, 10 days for $600.00
Operating Season: 6/20 to 8/31
Capacity: 150
Facilities: Cabins, Dorms
Camp's Comments: Open to visually impaired. Pool, horses, recreation, arts.
Visual Impairments

Marin YMCA Day Camp

1500 Los Gamos Road
San Rafael, CA 94903
Phone: 415/492-9622
Day Camp
Operator: Tim Byrd, 1500 Los Gamos Road, San Rafael, CA 94903 415/492-9622
Clientele/Fees: Coed from 5 to 12, 5 days for $103.00.
Operating Season: 6/15 to 8/30
General Physical Disabilities

Paivika

PO Box 3367
Crestline, CA 92325
Phone: 909/338-1102
Resident Camp
Director: Carolyn Hewitt
Operator: Crippled Children's Society, 7120 Franklin Ave., Los Angeles, CA 90046, 213/874-3300
Clientele/Fees: Coed from 7 to 65, 7 days for $630.00, 8 days for $720.00
Operating Season: 6/18 to 8/24
Capacity: 100
Facilities: Cabins
Camp's Comments: All facilities are wheelchair accessible.
General Physical Disabilities, Mobility Limitations

San Diego Youth Aquatics Ctr.

1750 Fiesta Island Road
San Diego, CA 92109-8402
Phone: 619/275-3384
Day Camp
Director: Elbert Buerger
Operator: Desert Pacific Council, 1207 Upas St., San Diego, CA 92103
Clientele/Fees: Boys from 8 to 18, Coed from 8 to 21, 5 days for $175.00, 2 days for $15.00, 1 day for $7.00, 10 days for $320.00
Operating Season: 7/4 to 8/15
Capacity: 200
Facilities: Tents, Other
Camp's Comments: Scout camp features aquatics, environment, health & safety.
General Physical Disabilities

Sproul Ranch "Deaf Kids Kamp"

PO Box 1109
Visalia, CA 93279-1109
Phone: 209/561-4935
Resident Camp
Director: Terry Sproul
Operator: PO Box 1109, Visalia, CA 93279-1109, 209/561-4935
Hearing Impairment

CONNECTICUT

Easter Seal Hemlocks Recreation Ctr

PO Box 198
Hebron, CT 06248-0198
Phone: 203/228-9496
Resident Camp
Director: Sunny P. Ku
Operator: Easter Seal Society of CT, PO Box 100, Hebron, CT 06248-0198, 203/228-9496

Clientele/Fees: Coed from 1 to 17, Adults from 18 to 59, Adults from 60 to 99, 11 days for $580.00, 11 days for $715.00
Operating Season: 6/11 to 8/18
Capacity: 120
Facilities: Cabins, Dorms, Lodge, Tents
Camp's Comments: Adaptive programs for special need populations.
General Physical Disabilities, Mobility Limitations

DELAWARE

Camp Manito

700 A. River Rd.
Wilmington, DE 19809
Phone: 302/764-2400
Day Camp
Director: William J. McCool III
Operator: United Cerebral Palsy of DE, 700 A. River Rd., Wilmington, DE 19809, 302/764-2400
Clientele/Fees: Coed from 3 to 25, 20 days for $150.00
Operating Season: 7/1 to 7/26
Capacity: 100
General Physical Disabilities

Children's Beach House

1800 Bay Avenue
Lewes, DE 19958
Phone: 302/645-9184
Resident Camp
Director: Harold L. Springer III
Operator: Children's Beach House Inc., 128A Senatorial Drive, Greenville Place, Wilmington, DE 19807, 302/655-4288
Clientele/Fees: Coed from 6 to 12, 31 days for $570.00
Operating Season: 6/14 to 8/15
Capacity: 23
Facilities: Dorms
Camp's Comments: DE residents only, communication and orthopedic handicapped.
General Physical Disabilities, Hearing Impairment

Lenape

Route 1, Box 58
Felton, DE 19943
Phone: 302/335-5626
Day Camp
Director: Patricia A. Preisen
Operator: U Cerebral Palsy of Del Inc., Route 1, Box 58, Felton, DE 19943, 302/335-5626
Clientele/Fees: Coed from 3 to 25, 20 days for $150.00, 10 days for $75.00
Operating Season: 7/6 to 7/31
Capacity: 60
Camp's Comments: Meets ADA standards for accessibility. A fun place to be!
General Physical Disabilities, Hearing Impairment, Visual Impairments

---

FLORIDA

Challenge

31600 Camp Challenge Rd
Sorrento, FL 32776
Phone: 904/383-4711
Day Camp, Resident Camp
Director: Jesse Shuman
Operator: Florida Easter Seals Society, 1010 Executive Drive Suite 231, Orlando, FL 32803, 407/896-7881
Clientele/Fees: Coed from 6 to 21, Adults from 21 to 90, 12 days for $590.00, 4 days for $125.00, 7 days for $300.00, 2 days for $75.00
Operating Season: 1/1 to 12/31
Facilities: Cabins, Dorms, Lodge
Camp's Comments: New wheelchair sports and asthma camps, open year-round.
General Physical Disabilities, Hearing Impairment, Mobility Limitations

IDAHO

Easter Seal East (ID)

Worley, ID 83873
Phone: 509/326-8292
Resident Camp
Operator: Easter Seal Society of WA, 17719 So Vaughn Rd, Vaughn, WA 98394 206/884-2722
Clientele/Fees: Coed from 7 to 18, Adults from 18 to 90, 7 days for $300.00
Operating Season: 6/15 to 8/2
Capacity: 50
Facilities: Cabins, Dorms
Camp's Comments: Quality outdoor recreation for disabled persons. *General Physical Disabilities, Mobility Limitations, Visual Impairments*

ILLINOIS

Camp Little Giant

Touch of Nature, Southern Illinois University
Carbondale, IL 62901-6623
Phone: 618/453-1121
Resident Camp
Director: Barbara Lanser, CTRS
Operator: Touch of Nature, SIUC, Carbondale, IL 62901-6623, 618/453-1121
Clientele/Fees: Coed from 6 to 60, 5 days for $340.00, 10 days for $525.00, 12 days for $640.00
Operating Season: 6/5 to 8/6
Capacity: 80
Facilities: Cabins, Dorms
Camp's Comments: Camping for children and adults with disabilities. *General Physical Disabilities, Hearing Impairment, Mobility Limitations, Visual Impairments*

Easter Seal Camp Heffernan

206 S Linden Suite 4A
Normal, IL 61761
Phone: 309/452-8074
Resident Camp
Director: David Bateman
Operator: Easter Seal Rehabilitation Ctr, 206 S Linden Suite 4A, Normal, IL 61761, 309/452-8074
Clientele/Fees: Coed from 6 to 20, 2 days for $40.00, 5 days for $250.00, 13 days for $450.00
Operating Season: 1/1 to 12/31
Facilities: Cabins, Tents, Lodge
Camp's Comments: Coed 6-Adults, Aul-to rent, 44 yrs. of service to disabled.
General Physical Disabilities, Mobility Limitations, Visual Impairments

Easter Seal Summer Camp (IL)

Hoover Outdoor Recreation Ctr
Yorkville, IL 60560
Phone: 312/896-1961
Resident Camp
Director: Richard N. Merz
Operator: Easter Seal Rehabilitation Ctr, 1230 N Highland Ave, Aurora, IL 60506, 708/896-1961
Clientele/Fees: Coed from 6 to 18, 7 days for $150.00
Operating Season: 7/27 to 8/3
Capacity: 35
Facilities: Cabins, Other
Camp's Comments: Non-residents of our service area fee for 7 days is $325.00
General Physical Disabilities, Mobility Limitations

Peacock Camp

38685 N Deep Lake Rd
Lake Villa, IL 60046
Phone: 708/356-5201

Resident Camp
Director: David & Peggy Bogenschutz
Operator: Peacock Camp Inc., 38685 N Deep Lake Rd, Lake Villa, IL 60046, 708/356-5201
Clientele/Fees: Boys from 13 to 17
Operating Season: 6/20 to 8/15
Capacity: 36
Facilities: Lodge
Camp's Comments: Peacock Camp serves 7-17 yr. olds w/orthopedic disabilities.
General Physical Disabilities, Hearing Impairment, Mobility Limitations

---

INDIANA

Bradford Woods Outdoor Ed & Camping Ctr-Camp Riley

5040 St. Road 67 North
Martinsville, IN 46151
Phone: 317/3422915
Resident Camp
Director: Gary M. Robb
Operator: Indiana University, Bradford Woods, 5040 St. Road 67 North, Martinsville, IN 46151
Clientele/Fees: Coed from 8 to 18, Adults from 28 to 70, 7 days for $300.00
Operating Season: 6/4 to 8/11
Capacity: 100
Facilities: Cabins, Dorms, Lodge, Tents, Teepees, Other
Camp's Comments: Serves children & adults w/disabilities. 20 mi. south of Indianapolis.
General Physical Disabilities, Mobility Limitations

Camp Millhouse

25600 Kelly Road
South Bend, IN 46614
Phone: 219/287-9833
Resident Camp

Sports, Everyone!

Director: Lea Pitcher
Operator: Camp Millhouse Inc., 3702 W Sample, South Bend, IN 46619, 219/233-2202
Clientele/Fees: Coed from 7 to 22, Adults from 22 to 70, 6 days for $250.00
Operating Season: 6/13 to 8/13
Capacity: 60
Facilities: Cabins
Camp's Comments: Serving the needs of persons w/disabilities for over 50 yrs.
General Physical Disabilities, Mobility Limitations

Happiness Bag Day Camp

1519 South 7th Street
Terre Haute, IN 47802
Phone: 812/234-8867
Day Camp
Director: Jodi A. Moan
Operator: Happiness Bag Inc., 1519 South 7th Street, Terre Haute, IN 47802, 812/234-8867
Clientele/Fees: Coed from 4 to 18, Adults from 18 +
Operating Season: 6/8 to 8/6
Capacity: 30
Camp's Comments: Serves developmentally disabled age 5-adult. $1.25 hr-9am-3.

General Physical Disabilities, Mobility Limitations

Isanogel

7601 W Isanogel Rd. 50-N
Muncie, IN 47304-9339
Phone: 317/288-1073
Resident Camp
Director: Vickie Strahan
Operator: Delaware Co. Easter Seal Society7601 W Isanogel Rd. 50-N, Muncie, IN 47304-9339, 317/288-1073
Clientele/Fees: Coed from 8 to 15, Adults from 16 to 25, Adults from 26 to, 6 days for $225, 12 days for $450.00.
Operating Season: 5/28 to 8/25
Capacity: 48

Facilities: Dorms
Camp's Comments: 30 years of camping for disabled children, teens & adults.
General Physical Disabilities, Hearing Impairment, Mobility Limitations, Visual Impairments

Twin Lakes Camp

15543 12th Road
Plymouth, IN 46563
Phone: 219/936-8320
Resident Camp
Director: Diana Parks
Operator: Southside Crippled Children's Aid/IN Easter Seal Society, 625 West Broadway, Mishawaka, IN 46545, 219/256-5949
Clientele/Fees: Coed from 7 to 26, Adults, 6 days for $225.00, 12 days for $450.00
Operating Season: 6/18 to 8/18
Capacity: 56
Facilities: Cabins
Camp's Comments: Program adapted to meet needs of campers stressing independence
General Physical Disabilities, Mobility Limitations

IOWA

Camp Courageous of Iowa

RR 2 PO Box 557
Monticello, IA 52310-0455
Phone: 319/465-5916
Resident Camp
Director: Jeanne Mullerleile, CCD
Operator: Camp Courageous of Iowa, RR 2 PO Box 557, Monticello, IA, 52310-0455, 319/465-5916
Clientele/Fees: Coed from 1 to 99, 6 days for $200.00
Operating Season: 1/1 to 12/31
Facilities: A-Frames, Cabins, Dorms, Lodge, Tents, Other
Camp's Comments: Yr-round camp for persons with disabilities adventure act.
General Physical Disabilities, Mobility Limitations

Easter Seal Camp Sunnyside

PO Box 4002
Des Moines, IA 50333
Phone: 515/289-1933
Day Camp, Resident Camp
Director: Martha Wittkowski
Operator: Easter Seal Society of Iowa, PO Box 4002, Des Moines, IA, 50333, 515/289-1933
Operating Season: 1/1 to 12/31
Capacity: 200
Facilities: Cabins, Lodge, Tents
Camp's Comments: Resident Camp 5/$360.00, 12/$720.00. Day Camp 5/$70.00
General Physical Disabilities, Mobility Limitations

KENTUCKY

Easter Seal KYSOC

1902 Easterday Rd.
Carrollron, KY 41008
Phone: 502/732-5333
Resident Camp
Director: C. Heidemann Miller
Operator: Kentucky Easter Seal Society, 233 East Broadway, Louisville, KY 40202-2007, 502/584-9781
Clientele/Fees: Coed from 6 to 21, Adults from 21 to 64, 6 days for $250.00, 12 days for $500.00
Operating Season: 5/25 to 8/9
Capacity: 150
Facilities: Cabins, Dorms
Camp's Comments: Rustic, small group living experience
General Physical Disabilities, Visual Impairments

LOUISIANA

LA Lions Camp for Handicapped & Diabetic Youth

PO Box 171
Leesville, LA 71496-0171
Phone: 318/239-0782
Resident Camp
Director: Raymond E. Cecil III, CCD
Operator: Louisiana Lions League, PO Box 171, Leesville, LA 71496-0171, 318/239-0782
Clientele/Fees: Coed from 8 to 19
Operating Season: 6/7 to 8/15
Capacity: 80
Facilities: Dorms
Camp's Comments: Camp for handicapped children and diabetic youth.
General Physical Disabilities, Hearing Impairment, Mobility Limitations, Visual Impairments

MARYLAND

Easter Seal Camp Fairlee Manor

22242 Bay Shore Rd
Chestertown, MD 21620
Phone: 410/778-0566
Day Camp, Resident Camp
Director: Michael Currence
Operator: Easter Seal Society of Del-Mar, 22242 Bay Shore Rd, Chestertown, MD 21620, 410/778-0566
Clientele/Fees: Coed from 5 to 14, Coed from 12 to 21, Adults from 21 to 95, 5 days for $700.00, 12 days for $1400.00
Operating Season: 6/16 to 8/16
Capacity: 120
Facilities: Cabins, Dorms
Camp's Comments: Summer camp & recreation programs for people w/disabilities.
General Physical Disabilities, Mobility Limitations, Visual Impairments

Greentop

Catoctin Mt Natl Park
15001 Park Central Road
Sabillasville, MD 21780
Phone: 301/293-0801
Resident Camp
Director: Cisco Nochera
Operator: The League: Serving people with disabilities, 1111 E Cold
Spring Lane, Baltimore, MD 21239, 301/323-0500
Clientele/Fees: Coed from 7 to 75, Adults from 36 to 75, 14 days for
$700.00, 7 days for $500.00
Operating Season: 6/26 to 8/13
Capacity: 70
Facilities: Cabins, Lodge, Tents
Camp's Comments: Physical handicaps and multiple handicaps 1 to 1
and 1 to 2.
General Physical Disabilities, Mobility Limitations

Melwood Recreation and Travel Center

Melwood Recreation and Travel Ctr
Nanjiemoy, MD 20662
Phone: 301/870-3226
Resident Camp
Director: Heidi Aldous
Operator: Melwood Farm, Rt. 1 Box 50-A, Nanjiemoy, MD 20662,
301/870-3226
Clientele/Fees: Coed from 14 to 69, Adults from, 54 to 69, 4 days for
$275.00, 5 days for $325.00, 7 days for $450.00
Operating Season: 1/1 to 12/31
Facilities: Cabins
Camp's Comments: Serves mentally disabled adults in year round
program.
General Physical Disabilities, Mobility Limitations

MICHIGAN

Ability

Easter Seals of Genesee Co., 1420 W Third Avenue
Flint, MI 48504-4897
Phone: 313/238-0475
Resident Camp
Director: Sally L. Walker
Operator: American Baptist Church of Michael, Baptist Camp, 2062
Ferns Rd., Lapeer, MI 48446, 517/332-3594
Clientele/Fees: Coed from 8 to 20, 5 days for $10.00
Operating Season: 6/21 to 8/15
Capacity: 30
Facilities: Cabins
Camp's Comments: All volunteer. Campers various disabilities, ages
8-20.
General Physical Disabilities

Camp Living Waters

Route 2 Box 73
Luther, MI 49656-9709
Phone: 616/797-5107
Resident Camp
Director: Brett Adler
Operator: Church of the United Brethren in Christ, Route 2 Box 73,
Luther, MI 49656-9709, 616/797-5107
Clientele/Fees: Coed from 8 to 17, Adults from 18 to 80, 5 days for
$159.00, 5 days for $174.00
Operating Season: 1/1 to 12/31
Capacity: 132
Facilities: A-Frames, Cabins, Tents, Teepees
Camp's Comments: Horseback Riding, Archery, Swimming, Canoe-
ing
General Physical Disabilities

137

Fowler Inc.

2315 Harmon Lake Road
Mayville, MI 48744
Phone: 517/673-2050
Resident Camp
Director: Stephen Greene
Operator: Camp Fowler Inc., 2315 Harmon Lake Road, Mayville, MI 48744, 517/673-2050
Clientele/Fees: Coed from 6 to 17, Adults from 18 to 60, 5 days for $310.00, 13 days for $600.00
Operating Season: 1/1 to 12/31
Capacity: 100
Facilities: Cabins, Lodge, Tents, Teepees
Camp's Comments: Yr-round camp for developmentally disabled persons.
General Physical Disabilities, Hearing Impairment, Visual Impairments

Indian Trails Camp Inc.

0-1859 Lake Michigan Drive
Grand Rapids, MI 49504
Phone: 616/677-5251
Resident Camp
Director: Lynn Gust
Operator: Indian Trails Camp Inc., 0185 Lake Michigan Drive, Grand Rapids, MI 49504, 616/677-5251
Clientele/Fees: Coed from 6-25, Adults from 26 to 70, 6 days for $354.00, 10 days for $590.00, 12 days for $708.00
Operating Season: 6/18 to 8/18
Capacity: 75
Facilities: Cabins
Camp's Comments: Camp for physically impaired children and adults.
General Physical Disabilities, Mobility Limitations

Shady Trails Camp

PO Box 500
Northport, MI 49670
Phone: 616/386-5111
Resident Camp
Director: Joanne Pierson, MS, CCC-S
Operator: Holly K. Craig Ph.D., University of Michigan Communicative Disorders Clinic,1111 East Catherine, Ann Arbor, MI 48109, 313/764-8442
Clientele/Fees: Coed from 5 to 17, 14 days for $1275.00, 21 days for $2200.00
Operating Season: 6/26 to 7/29
Capacity: 132
Facilities: Cabins
Camp's Comments: Intensive speech-language therapy camp on Grand Traverse Bay
Hearing Impairment

Echo Grove Salvation Army Camp

1101 Camp Rd
Leonard, MI 48036
Phone: 313/628-3108
Resident Camp
Director: Harold Campbell
Operator: The Salvation Army, 1101 Camp Rd, Leonard, MI 48367, 313/628-3108
Clientele/Fees: Boys from 7 to 11, Girls from 7 to 11, Coed from 7 to 14, Adults from 55 to
Operating Season: 6/15 to 8/15
Facilities: Cabins, Dorms, Lodge
Camp's Comments: Summer camp fees are based on income. Yr-round rentals available.
Visual Impairments

MINNESOTA

Camp New Hope Inc.

HCR 3 Box 578
McGregor, MN 55760
Phone: 218/426-3560
Resident Camp
Director: Barbara Dargatz
Operator: Barbara Dargatz and Board, HCR 3 Box 578, McGregor, MN 55760, 218/426-3560
Clientele/Fees: Coed from 5 to 18, Adults from 18 to 99, 5 days for $280.00
Operating Season: 6/1 to 8/31
Capacity: 48
Facilities: Cabins, Other, Lodge, Tents
Camp's Comments: Serving individuals with developmental disabilities & physical challenges.
General Physical Disabilities, Mobility Limitations

Courage

8046 83rd St. NW
Maple Lake, MN 55358
Phone: 612/963-3121
Resident Camp
Director: Roger Upcraft
Operator: Courage Center, 3915 Golden Valley Rd, Golden Valley, MN 55422, 612/520-0504
Clientele/Fees: Coed from 7 to 18, Adults from 18 to 45, Adults from 45 to 90
Operating Season: 6/15 to 9/1
Capacity: 145
Facilities: Cabins, Dorms, Lodge, Tents
Camp's Comments: Resident program. Physical disability, cancer - child & adult.
General Physical Disabilities, Hearing Impairment, Visual Impairments

Courage North

Lake George, MN 56458
Phone: 218/266-3658
Resident Camp
Director: Thomas Fogarty
Operator: Courage Center, 3915 Golden Valley Rd., Golden Valley, MN 55422, 612/520-0504
Clientele/Fees: Coed from 8 to 17, Adults from 18 to 65, Adults from 65 to 99
Operating Season: 6/15 to 9/1
Camp's Comments: Program for physically handicap-burn camp-hearing impaired
General Physical Disabilities, Hearing Impairment, Mobility Limitations, Visual Impairments

Friendship

10509 108th St. NW
Annandale, MN 55302
Phone: 612/274-8376
Resident Camp
Director: Georgann Rumsey
Operator: Friendship Ventures,10509 108th St. NW, Annandale, MN 55302, 612/274-8376
Clientele/Fees: Coed from 5 to 80, 2 days for $165.00, 6 days for $345.00, 14 days for $855.00
Operating Season: 6/1 to 9/1
Capacity: 130
Facilities: Cabins, Lodge, Other
Camp's Comments: Services for children & adults w/disabilities. Travel program.
General Physical Disabilities, Mobility Limitations

Knutson

Manhattan Beach, MN 56463
Phone: 218/543-4232
Resident Camp
Director: Robert Larson

Sports, Everyone!

Operator: Lutheran Social Service of MN, Camp Knutson, 2029 South 6th #106, Brainerd, MN 56401 218/829-9214
Clientele/Fees: Coed from 1 to 18, Adults from 19 to 64, Adults from 64 to 75, 6 days for $210
Operating Season: 5/15 to 9/30
Capacity: 72
Facilities: Cabins, Dorms
Camp's Comments: Group camping for handicapped populations
Hearing Impairment

SKIP Camp Family Retreat, Inc.

11208 Minnetonka Mills Rd.
Maple Lake, MN 55343
Phone: 612/935-5581
Day Camp, Resident Camp
Director: Barb Donaghy
Operator: SKIP Camp Family Retreat Inc., 11208 Minnetonka Mills Rd., Maple Lake, MN 55343, 612/935-5581
Clientele/Fees: Coed from 5 to 21, Adults
Operating Season: 8/18 to 8/23
Capacity: 120
Facilities: Cabins, Dorms
Camp's Comments: For children on life support equipment and their families
General Physical Disabilities, Hearing Impairment

MISSISSIPI

Tik-A-Witha

PO Box 126
Van Fleet, MS 38877
Phone: 601/447-3250
Resident Camp
Director: Julia L. Newsom
Operator: Prairie GS Council Inc., PO Box 1087, Tupelo, MS 38802, 601/844-7577
Clientele/Fees: Girls from 7 to 17, 6 days for $100.00, 13 days for $200.00
Operating Season: 6/12 to 8/7

142

Capacity: 150
Facilities: Cabins, Tents, Lodge
Camp's Comments: Open to all girls, one week for handicapped children
General Physical Disabilities, Mobility Limitations

MISSOURI

Wonderland Camp Foundation

PO Box 1089
Rocky Mount, MO 65072
Phone: 314/392-1000
Resident Camp
Director: Cari Williams
Operator: Allen R. Moore, PO Box 1089, Rocky Mount, MO 65072, 314/392-1000
Clientele/Fees: Coed from 6 to 99, Adults from 6 to 99, 7 days for $250.00
Operating Season: 5/30 to 9/25
Capacity: 153
Facilities: Cabins
Camp's Comments: We are a camp that serve the mentally and physically disabled.
General Physical Disabilities

NEBRASKA

Camp Easter Seal (NE)

Rt 1 Box 51B1
Milford, NE 68405
Phone: 402/761-2875
Resident Camp
Director: Andi Reed
Operator: The Nebraska Easter Seal Society, 12100 W Center Rd. #820, Omaha, NE 68144, 402/571-2162
Clientele/Fees: Coed, 5 days for $425.00
Operating Season: 6/4 to 8/11

Sports, Everyone!
Capacity: 50
Facilities: Cabins, Lodge
Camp's Comments: Accessible facility and program for people with disabilities.
General Physical Disabilities

Camp Allen Inc. for Individuals with Disabilities

56 Camp Allen Road
Bedford, NH 03110-6606
Phone: 603/622-8471
Resident Camp
Director: Lori A. Stumpfol
Operator: Boston Kiwanis/Manchester Lions Clubs, 56 Camp Allen Road, Bedford, NH, 03110-6606, 603/622-8471
Clientele/Fees: Boys from 5 to 18, Girls from 5 to 18, Adults from 18 to 60, Adults from 60 to 90, 7 days for $430.00, 12 days for $740.00
Operating Season: 6/18 to 8/20
Capacity: 330
Facilities: Cabins, Dorms
Camp's Comments: Individ. 5-90 w/disabilities: arts/nature/aquatics/overnite camp.
General Physical Disabilities, Hearing Impairment, Visual Impairments

Jotoni Camp

51 Old Stirling Road
Warren, NJ 07059-5809
Phone: 908/753-4244
Day Camp, Resident Camp
Director: Richard Rowe
Operator: ARC of Somerset, 141 S Main St., Manville, NJ, 08835, 908/725 8544

Clientele/Fees: Coed from 5 to 21, 5 days for $50.00, 7 days for $200.00
Operating Season: 7/1 to 8/19
Capacity: 100
Facilities: Cabins
Camp's Comments: Campers with mental retardation and some physically handicapped.
General Physical Disabilities

Merry Heart/Easter Seal

RD #2 O'Brien Rd
Hackettstown, NJ 07840
Phone: 908/852-3896
Day Camp, Resident Camp
Director: Mary Ellen Ross, CCD
Operator: Easter Seal Society of NJ, RD #2 O'Brien Rd, Hackettstown, NJ 07840, 908/852-3896
Clientele/Fees: Coed from 5 to 17, Adults from 18 to 60, Adults from 61 to 90, 6 days for $400.00, 12 days for $650.00, 6 days for $500.00, 10 days for $700.00
Operating Season: 6/10 to 8/33
Capacity: 125
Facilities: Cabins
Camp's Comments: Programs for special populations, mainstreaming non-disabled
General Physical Disabilities

NEW MEXICO

Easter Seal Camp (NM)

General Delivery
Vanderwagen, NM 87326
Phone: 505/778-5796
Resident Camp
Director: Mark Herrell
Operator: Easter Seal Society of New Mexico, 2819 Richmond Drive NE, Albuquerque, NM 87107, 505/888-3811
Clientele/Fees: Boys, Girls, Coed, Adults, 6 days for $400.00, 7 days

for $425.00, 10 days for $450.00
Operating Season: 6/11 to 7/31
Capacity: 40
Facilities: Dorms, Lodge
Camp's Comments: Traditional camping-wilderness setting-disabled & non-disabled
General Physical Disabilities, Mobility Limitations, Visual Impairments

NEW YORK

Clover Patch Camp

PO Box 2669 Helping Hand Lane
Glenville, NY 12325-2669
Phone: 518/399-8124
Resident Camp
Director: Lori Hoefer
Operator: United Cerebral Palsy Assn., PO Box 2669 Helping Hand Lane, Glenville, NY 12325-2669, 518/399-8124
Clientele/Fees: Coed from 4 to 26, 13 days for $675.00, 13 days for $925.00
Operating Season: 7/3 to 8/20
Capacity: 45
Facilities: Cabins
Camp's Comments: Qualified staff gives caring camping experience to disabled.
General Physical Disabilities, Mobility Limitations

Mid-Hudson Valley Camp

PO 197
Esopus, NY 12429
Phone: 914/384-6620
Resident Camp
Director: Leo Forrest
Operator: Marist Brothers, PO Box 197, Esopus, NY 12429, 914/384-6620
Clientele/Fees: Boys from 13 to 15, Coed from 5 to 18, Adults from 18 to 65, 7 days for $160.00, 12 days for $385.00

Operating Season: 6/17 to 10/1
Capacity: 85
Facilities: Dorms
Camp's Comments: Serves special people: deaf, retarded & children with cancer.
Hearing Impairment, Mobility Limitations

West Side YMCA

5 West 63rd Street
New York, NY 10023
Phone: 212/875-4112
Day Camp
Director: Ravenell Williams
Operator: 5 West 63rd Street, New York, NY, 10023, 212/875-4112
Clientele/Fees: Coed, 10 days for $265.00
Operating Season: 6/19 to 8/25
Capacity: 400
Camp's Comments: West Side YMCA primary goal is to provide fun in safe envir.
General Physical Disabilities

NORTH CAROLINA

Easter Seal Camping Program (NC)

Easter Seal Society of NC
2315 Myron Drive
Raleigh, NC 27607-3344
Phone: 919/783-8898
Resident Camp
Director: Karen A. Hamilton
Operator: Easter Seal Society of NC, 2315 Myron Drive, Raleigh, NC 27607-3344, 919/783-8898
Clientele/Fees: Coed from 7 to 18, Adults from 19 to 54, Adults from 55 to, 6 days for $295.00
Operating Season: 6/7 to 7/10
Capacity: 40
Facilities: Cabins
Camp's Comments: Emphasis—Mainstreaming for campers w/dis-

abilities.
General Physical Disabilities, Mobility Limitations, Visual Impairments

---

OHIO

Allyn

1414 Lake Allyn Road
Batavia, OH 45103
Phone: 513/732-0240
Resident Camp
Director: Irene K. Taylor
Operator: Stepping Stone Center, 5650 Given Rd, Cincinnati, OH 45243, 513/831-4660
Clientele/Fees: Coeds from 7 to 65, 6 days for $280.00, 12 days for $565.00
Operating Season: 5/7 to 9/15
Capacity: 69
Facilities: Cabins
Camp's Comments: A camp for children and adults with disabilities.
General Physical Disabilities

CHAMP Camp

11001 Buckeye Rd.
Cleveland, OH 44104
Phone: 216/795-7100
Day Camp
Director: David Mable
Operator: Achievement Ctr for Children, 15000 Cheerful Lane, Strongsville, OH 44136, 216/238-6200
Clientele/Fees: Coed from 4 to 12, 15 days for $20
Operating Season: 6/15 to 8/15
Capacity: 40
Camp's Comments: Inclusive recreation program for many abilities.
General Physical Disabilities, Mobility Limitations, Visual Impairments

Cheerful

15000 Cheerful Lane
Strongsville, OH 44136
Phone: 216/238-6200
Resident Camp
Director: David Mable
Operator: Achievement Ctr for Children, 15000 Cheerful Lane, Strongsville, OH 44136, 216/238-6200
Clientele/Fees: Coed from 5 to 65, 1 day for $45.00
Operating Season: 6/15 to 8/17
Capacity: 50
Facilities: Cabins, Teepees
Camp's Comments: Physical disabilities/speech; integrated children's session.
General Physical Disabilities

Echoing Hills

36272 C R 79
Warsaw, OH 43844-9990
Phone: 614/327-2311
Resident Camp
Director: Shaker Samuel
Operator: Echoing Hills Village Inc., 36272 C R 79, Warsaw, OH 43844-9990, 614/327-2311
Clientele/Fees: Coed from 7 to 70, Adults from 7 to 70, 5 days for $230.00, 6 days for $270.00, 7 days for $310.00
Operating Season: 6/15 to 8/17
Capacity: 100
Facilities: Cabins, Dorms, Lodge
Camp's Comments: Camp for special population & developmentally disabled.
General Physical Disabilities, Mobility Limitations, Visual Impairments

Emanuel-Day

2321 Rugby Rd.
Dayton, OH 45406

Phone: 513/274-3084
Day Camp
Director: Nancy Crawford
Operator: Camp Emanuel Board of Directors
Clientele/Fees: Coed from 4 to 14, 5 days for $60.00, 10 days for $110.00, 15 days for $165.00
Operating Season: 6/19 to 6/30
Facilities: Lodge
Camp's Comments: For hearing impaired and normal hearing youth.
Hearing Impairment

Happiness at St. Augustine Academy

14808 Lake Avenue
Lakewood, OH 44107
Phone: 216/696-6525
Day Camp
Director: William Tighe
Operator: Apostolate for Persons with Developmental Disabilities, 1031 Superior Ave. Rm. 331, Cleveland, OH 44114, 216/696-6525
Clientele/Fees: Coed from 6 to 21, 5 days for $85.00
Operating Season: 6/17 to 7/26
Camp's Comments: Serves persons with developmental disabilities.
Mobility Limitations

Highbrook Lodge

12944 Aquilla Road
Chardon, OH 44024
Phone: 216/286-3121
Resident Camp
Director: Bashir Masoodi
Operator: Cleveland Society For Blind, 1909 E 101st St., Cleveland, OH 44106-4110, 216/791-8118
Clientele/Fees: Coed from 2 to 17, Adults from 18 to 65, Adults from 65 to 92, 3 days for $25.00, 7 days for $70.00, 10 days for $350.00
Operating Season: 6/14 to 8/18
Facilities: Dorms, Lodge
Hearing Impairment, Visual Impairments

Stepping Stone

5650 Given Road
Cincinnati, OH 45243
Phone: 513/831-4660
Day Camp
Director: Dennis D. Carter
Operator: Stepping Stones Center for Handicapped, 5650 Given Road, Cincinnati, OH 45243, 513/831-4660
Operating Season: 6/00 to 8/19
Capacity: 200
Camp's Comments: Nonprofit United Way fees on sliding scale all disabilities.
General Physical Disabilities

OREGON

Camp Easter Seal (OR)

Boat Route, North Lake
Lakeside, OR 97405
Phone: 503/344-2247
Resident Camp
Director: Diane Battaglia, CTRS
Operator: Easter Seal Society of Oregon, 3575 Donald St. Eugene, OR 97405, 503/344-2247
Clientele/Fees: Coed from 6 to 99, 6 days for $250.00
Operating Season: 6/18 to 9/1
Capacity: 42
Facilities: Cabins, Lodge
Camp's Comments: For campers with & without disabilities. Challenge/independence.
General Physical Disabilities, Mobility Limitations

Camp Taloali Inc.

15934 North Santian Hwy
Stayton, OR 97449
Phone: 503/769-6415

Resident Camp
Director: George Scheler
Operator: George Scheler, 4738 El Cedro Loop NE, Salem, OR 97305, 800/735-2900
Clientele/Fees: Coed from 9 to 18, 6 days for $145.00
Operating Season: 8/1 to 8/28
Capacity: 100
Facilities: Cabins
Camp's Comments: Deaf owned and operated; serves deaf children
Hearing Impairment

Evans Creek/Upward Bound Camp

36155 North Fork Road
Lyons, OR 97358
Phone: 503/897-2447
Resident Camp
Director: Jerry & Laura Pierce
Operator: Jerry Pierce, 36155 North Fork Road, Lyons, OR 97358, 503/897-2447
Clientele/Fees: Coed from 12 to 99, 5 days for $215.00
Operating Season: 1/1 to 12/31
Capacity: 50
Facilities: Cabins, Dorms, Lodge
Camp's Comments: Trained staff serve needs of persons with disabilities.
General Physical Disabilities, Visual Impairments

Meadowood Springs Speech and Hearing Camp

Rt. 1 Box 48
Weston, OR 97886
Phone: 503/566-2191
Resident Camp
Director: Albert R. Jacques, Executive Director
Operator: Diana Gorham, Camp Director, PO Box 1925, Pendleton, OR 97801-0030, 503/276-2752
Clientele/Fees: Coed from 6 to 16
Operating Season: 6/15 to 8/15
Capacity: 250

Facilities: A-Frames, Cabins, Dorms, Lodge
Camp's Comments: Speech and hearing therapy, individual or group.
Hearing Impairment

Mt. Hood Kiwanis Camp Inc.

PO Box 206
Rhododendron, OR 97049
Phone: 503/272-3288
Resident Camp
Director: Gene Nudelman
Operator: Mt. Hood Kiwanis Camp, 9320 SW Barbar Blvd Suite, Portland, OR 97217, 503/452-7416
Clientele/Fees: Coed from 9 to 35, 6 days for $275.00, 3 days for $120.00
Operating Season: 6/18 to 8/11
Capacity: 120
Facilities: Dorms, Lodge
Camp's Comments: Recreation & education for people with disabilities.
General Physical Disabilities

PENNSYLVANIA

AIM

51 McMurray Rd.
Pittsburgh, PA 15241
Phone: 412/833-5600
Day Camp
Director: Martin P. Brocco
Operator: South Hills YMCA, 51 McMurray Rd., Pittsburgh, PA 15241, 412/833-5600
Clientele/Fees: Coed from 3 to 21, 10 days for $85.00
Operating Season: 6/30 to 8/31
Capacity: 150
General Physical Disabilities, Mobility Limitations

Camp Can-Do

Easter Seal Society
PO Box 333
Kulpsville, PA 19443
Phone: 215/368-7000
Day Camp
Director: Janet B. Rubien
Operator: Easter Seal Society, 468 N Middletown Road, Media, PA 19063, 215/256-4211
Clientele/Fees: Coed from 3 to 25, 5 days for $105.00, 29 days for $630.00
Operating Season: 7/1 to 8/9
Capacity: 45
Camp's Comments: Specialized day camp, transportation cost included.
General Physical Disabilities, Mobility Limitations

Camp Dumore

Easter Seal Society
468 N Middletown Road
Media, PA 19063
Phone: 215/565-2353
Day Camp
Director: Janet B. Rubien
Operator: Easter Seal Society, 468 N Middletown Road, Media, PA 19063, 215/565-2353
Clientele/Fees: Coed from 3 to 25, 5 days for $105.00, 29 days for $630.00
Operating Season: 7/2 to 8/10
Capacity: 40
Camp's Comments: Specialized day camp. Transportation prices included.
General Physical Disabilities, Mobility Limitations

Camp Surefoot

Easter Seal Society
2400 Trenton Rd.

Levittown, PA 19056
Phone: 215/565-2353
Day Camp
Director: Janet B. Rubien
Operator: Easter Seal Society, 468 N Middletown Road, Media, PA 19063, 215/945-1730
Clientele/Fees: Coed from 3 to 25, 5 days for $105.00, 29 days for $630.00
Operating Season: 7/1 to 8/9
Capacity: 60
Camp's Comments: Specialized day camp. Transportation prices included.
General Physical Disabilities, Mobility Limitations

Carefree

Easter Seal Society
1525 E Lincoln Highway
Coatesville, PA 19320
Phone: 215/363-4552
Day Camp
Director: Janet B. Rubien
Operator: Easter Seal Society, 468 N Middletown Road, Media, PA 19063, 215/383-4552
Clientele/Fees: Coed from 3 to 25, 5 days for $105.00, 29 days for $630.00
Operating Season: 7/8 to 8/11
Facilities: Lodge
Camp's Comments: Day camp for the disabled. Transportation cost included.
General Physical Disabilities

Make-a-Friend

Easter Seal Society
3975 Conshohocken Avenue
Philadelphia, PA 19131
Phone: 215/879-1000
Day Camp
Director: Janet B. Rubien
Operator: Easter Seal Society, 468 N Middletown Road, Media, PA 19063, 215/879-1000

Sports, Everyone!

Clientele/Fees: Coed from 3 to 21, 15 days for $345.00, 15 days for $195.00, 29 days for $630.00
Operating Season: 7/1 to 8/9
Capacity: 50
Camp's Comments: Specialized day camp. $115 with transportation, $65 without.
General Physical Disabilities, Mobility Limitations

Samuel Thompson Scout Camp

Elwyn, Inc.
Elwyn, PA 19063
Phone: 215/891-2299
Day Camp
Director: Jim Marenger
Operator: Elwyn Institutes, Elwyn, PA 19063, 215/891-2302
Clientele/Fees: Boys from 10 to 70, Girls from 10 to 50
Operating Season: 6/20 to 8/31
Capacity: 24
Facilities: Tents
Camp's Comments: Camp is one part program offered to our residents
Hearing Impairment

Variety Club Camp and Developmental Center

Valley Forge & Potshop Rds., Box 609
Worcester, PA 19490
Phone: 215/584-4366
Day Camp
Director: A. Doloff & R. McLemore
Operator: Variety Club of Philadelphia Inc., Box 609, Valley Forge & Potshop Rds., Worcester, PA 19490, 215/584-4366
Clientele/Fees: Coed from 7 to 18
Operating Season: 6/25 to 8/19
Capacity: 225
Facilities: Cabins
Camp's Comments: A year-round facility serving children with disabilities
General Physical Disabilities, Hearing Impairment, Mobility Limitations

156

SOUTH CAROLINA

Burnt Gin Camp

Wedgefield, SC 29168
Phone: 803/494-3145
Resident Camp
Director: Marie Aimone
Operator: Dir. of Children's Rehabilitative Services, DHEC/CRS Box 101106, Columbia, SC 29211, 803/737-4050
Clientele/Fees: Coed, 7 to 15
Operating Season: 6/10 to 8/9
Capacity: 80
Facilities: Cabins
Camp's Comments: A camp for children with special health care needs.
General Physical Disabilities, Hearing Impairment, Mobility Limitations

Clemson Univ. Outdoor Lab

263 Lehotsky Hall
Clemson, SC 29634-1005
Phone: 803/646-7502
Resident Camp
Director: Charlie R. White
Operator: Clemson University 263 Lehotsky Hall, Clemson, SC 29634-1005, 803/646-7502
Clientele/Fees: Coed from 8 to 60
Operating Season: 6/10 to 8/15
Capacity: 150
Facilities: Cabins
Camp's Comments: Conference Center Complex; during non-summer months.
Hearing Impairment, Visual Impairments

TENNESSEE

Camp Discovery

400 Camp Discovery Dr.
Gainesboro, TN 38562
Phone: 615/268-0239
Resident Camp
Director: David Casey
Operator: Tennessee Jaycee Fund Inc., 701 E 4th St., Chattanooga, TN 37403, 615/267-9718
Clientele/Fees: Coed from 6 to 99, Adults from 6 to 99, 5 days from $150.00
Operating Season: 6/1 to 8/30
Capacity: 30
Facilities: Dorms
Camp's Comments: Mentally, emotionally, and/or physically handicapped.
General Physical Disabilities

Camp Easter Seal (TN)

6300 Benders Ferry Road
Mt. Juliet, TN 37122
Phone: 615/444-2829
Resident Camp
Director: Ron Sanders
Operator: Easter Seal Society of Tennessee Inc., 2001 Woodmont Blvd, Nashville, TN 37215 615/292-6640
Clientele/Fees: Coed from 6 to 25, Adults from 25 to 99, 6 days for $235.00
Operating Season: 6/9 to 8/4
Capacity: 72
Facilities: Cabins, Lodge
General Physical Disabilities

Clyde M. York 4-H Center

Rt. 13 Box 237 Pomona Rd.
Crossville, TN 38555-8527

Phone: 615/788-2288
Resident Camp
Director: Conrad John Welch
Operator: University of Tennessee, Rt. 13 Box 237, Pomona Rd., Crossville, TN 38555-8527, 615/788-2288
Clientele/Fees: Coed from 9 to 19, Adults from 18 to 99, 5 days for $63.00
Operating Season: 5/30 to 8/20
Capacity: 404
Facilities: Dorms, Lodge, Tents
General Physical Disabilities

TEXAS

Camp C.A.M.P.

PO Box 999
Center Point, TX 78010
Phone: 210/634-2267
Resident Camp
Director: Shelley T. Watanabe
Operator: Camp Children's Association for Maximum Potential, PO Box 27086, San Antonio, TX, 78227, 210/671-2598
Clientele/Fees: Coed from 5 to 22, 6 days for $340.00
Operating Season: 6/6 to 8/15
Capacity: 275
Facilities: Cabins, Dorms
Camp's Comments: Primarily serves population not otherwise served & siblings.
General Physical Disabilities

Camp Summit

Route 1 Box 191 A
Argyle, TX 76226
Phone: 817/455-2213
Resident Camp
Director: Jeff Guidry
Operator: Camp Summit Inc., 2915 LBJ Freeway, Suite #183, Dallas, TX 75234-7607, 214/484-8900

Sports, Everyone!

Clientele/Fees: Coed from 6 to 99, 6 days for $265.00
Operating Season: 5/28 to 8/18
Capacity: 64
Facilities: Cabins
Camp's Comments: Camp Summit serves all disabilities regardless of type.
General Physical Disabilities, Hearing Impairment, Visual Impairments

Texas Elks Camp

Rt. 5 Box 185
Gonzales, TX 78629-9613
Phone: 210/672-7561
Resident Camp
Director: Leroy H. Haverlah, Jr.
Operator: Texas Elks Camp, Rt. 5 Box 185, Gonzales, TX 78629-9613, 210/672-7561
Clientele/Fees: Coed, 6 to 16
Operating Season: 6/18 to 8/5
Capacity: 168
Facilities: Lodge, Tents
Camp's Comments: Therapeutic fun for TX kids w/disabilities, including burns.
Hearing Impairment, Mobility Limitations

Texas Lions Camp

PO Box 247
Kerrville, TX 78029-0247
Phone: 210/896-8500
Resident Camp
Director: Dwight Evans
Operator: Texas Lions League, PO Box 247, Kerrville, TX 78029-0247, 210/896-8500
Clientele/Fees: Coed from 7 to 17
Operating Season: 6/5 to 8/13
Capacity: 400
Facilities: Dorms
Camp's Comments: Free camps for physically handicapped and diabetic children.
Hearing Impairment, Mobility Limitations, Visual Impairments

UTAH

Camp Kostopulos

2500 Emigration Canyon
Salt Lake City, UT 84108
Phone: 801/582-0700
Day Camp, Resident Camp
Director: Gary Ethington
Operator: Camp Kostopulos, 2500 Emigration Canyon, Salt Lake City, UT 84108, 801/582-0700
Clientele/Fees: Coed from 3 to 99, Adults from 30 to 99, 5 days for $245.00, 5 days for $275.00, 5 days for $295.00, 5 days for $350.00
Operating Season: 6/14 to 8/30
Capacity: 50
Facilities: Cabins, Tents
Camp's Comments: A camp for persons w/special needs. All ages & disabilities.
General Physical Disabilities, Hearing Impairment, Mobility Limitations

VIRGINIA

Easter Seal–East (VA)

Rt. 1 Box 111
Milford, VA 22514
Phone: 804/633-9855
Resident Camp
Director: Devin Brown
Operator: Virginia Easter Seal Society, PO Box 5496, Roanoke, VA 24012, 703/362-1656
Clientele/Fees: Coed from 5 to 17, Adults from 18 to 80, 6 days for $450.00 12 days for $900.00
Operating Season: 6/1 to 8/17
Capacity: 38
Facilities: Lodge
Camp's Comments: For children & adults with physical and mental disabilities
General Physical Disabilities, Hearing Impairment, Visual Impairments

Easter Seal–West (VA)

Rt. 2
New Castle, VA 24127
Phone: 703/362-1656
Resident Camp
Director: Cid Chatfield
Operator: Easter Seal Society of VA, Inc., 4841 Williamson Rd. PO Box 5496, Roanoke, VA 24021, 703/362-1656
Clientele/Fees: Coed from 5 to 17, Adults from 18 to 80, 6 days for $490.00, 12 days for $980.00, 29 days for $2250.00
Operating Season: 6/1 to 8/20
Capacity: 85
Facilities: Cabins
Camp's Comments: Serves children/adults with MR, physical and speech disability.
General Physical Disabilities, Hearing Impairment, Visual Impairments

WASHINGTON

Burton

9326 SW Bayview Drive
Vashon Island, WA 98070
Phone: 206/463-2512
Resident Camp
Director: Tom Nielsen
Operator: American Baptist Churches of the N.W., 9326 SW Bayview Drive, Vashon Island, WA 98070, 206/463-2512
Clientele/Fees: Coed from 7 to 10, Coed from 11 to 13, Coed from 14 to 15, Coed from 16 to 18, 6 days for $155.00
Operating Season: 6/15 to 9/8
Capacity: 200
Facilities: Cabins
Camp's Comments: Camps for religious ed, music & developmentally disabled.
Hearing Impairment

Easter Seal–West (WA)

PO Box J
Vaughn, WA 98394
Phone: 206/884-2722
Resident Camp
Director: Bill McIntyre
Operator: Easter Seal Society of WA, PO Box J, Vaughn, WA 98394, 206/884-2722
Clientele/Fees: Coed from 9 to 18, Adults from 18 to 65, Adults from 65 to 90, 7 days for $300.00, 5 days for $275.00, 4 days for $250.00
Operating Season: 6/13 to 9/18
Capacity: 50
Facilities: Dorms, A-Frames
Camp's Comments: Trip camping for children/adults all ages with disabilities.
General Physical Disabilities, Mobility Limitations, Visual Impairments

WISCONSIN

Easter Seal Center for Camping & Recreation

N9888, Hwy. 13 N
Wisconsin Dells, WI 53965
Phone: 608/254-8319
Resident Camp
Director: Kenneth H. Saville
Operator: Easter Seal Society of Wisconsin, 101 Nob Hill Rd., Madison, WI 53713-2149, 608/254-8319
Clientele/Fees: Coed from 8 to 17, Adults, 6 days for $265.00, 12 days for $525.00
Operating Season: 6/10 to 8/5
Capacity: 127
Facilities: Cabins, Dorms, Lodge, Tents
Camp's Comments: Nature trails. 400 acres. Wheelchair accessible.
General Physical Disabilities, Mobility Limitations

Wisconsin Badger Camp

Rt. 2 Box 351
Prairie Du Chien, WI 53821
Phone: 608/988-4558
Resident Camp
Director: Brent Bowers
Operator: Wisconsin Badger Camp, Box 240, Platteville, WI 52818, 608/348-9689
Clientele/Fees: Coed from 3 to 93, Adults, 6 days for $235.00, 13 days for $525.00
Operating Season: 6/1 to 8/18
Capacity: 80
Facilities: Dorms, Lodge, Tents
Camp's Comments: Accepts any individual who is developmentally challenged.
General Physical Disabilities

Wisconsin Lions Camp

46 County A
Rosholt, WI 54473
Phone: 715/677-4761
Resident Camp
Director: Tony Omernik, CCD
Operator: Wisconsin Lions Camp, 46 County A, WI 54473, 715/677-4761
Clientele/Fees: Coed from 6 to 18, Adults
Operating Season: 6/1 to 8/30
Capacity: 200
Facilities: Cabins, Lodge
Camp's Comments: Program serves visually/hearing/mentally impaired children only.
Hearing Impairment, Visual Impairments

Travel and Tourism

Following are some pointers for visiting national parks and other sites. Be sure to contact the parks and attractions when planning a visit for the most up-to-date information.

Golden Access Passport for Persons Who are Blind or Permanently Disabled

The Golden Access Passport is a lifetime entrance pass to those national parks, monuments, historic sites, recreation areas, and national wildlife refuges that charge a LWCFA (Land and Water Conservation Fund Act) entrance fee.

The Golden Access Passport admits the pass holder and any accompanying passengers in a private vehicle. Where entry is not by private vehicle, the passport admits the pass holder, spouse, and children.

The Golden Access Passport also provides a 50% discount on federal LWCFA use fees charged for facilities and services such as camping, swimming, parking, boat launching, and cave tours. In some cases where use fees are charged, only the pass holder will be given the 50% reduction; for example, cave tours, elevator services, or group camping. Unlike the Golden Age Passport, it does not cover or reduce special recreation permit fees or fees charged by concessioners.

A Golden Access Passport may be obtained at any federal area where a LWCFA entrance fee is charged or at a park agency (but not yet through the mail). To find the agency nearest to you, contact the Office of Public Inquires of the National Park Service at the following address:

Office of Public Inquiries, Room 1013
U.S. Department of the Interior
1849 C Street, NW
P.O. Box 37127
Washington DC 20013-7127

The Golden Access Passport is available only to citizens or permanent residents of the United States, regardless of age, who have been medically determined to be blind or permanently disabled. A passport may be obtained by showing proof of medically determined blindness or permanent disability and eligibility for receiving benefits under federal law.

Visiting the National Parks

Because each location is different, individual parks should be contacted for information on special accommodations for the disabled. Some of the larger parks and monuments—Yosemite, the Grand Canyon, and the Statue of Liberty, for example—have wheelchairs for loan to individuals. (A wheelchair rental concession has also been proposed for the Washington DC Mall area.) Some parks may have accommodations for the visually impaired, such as Braille brochures or audiotapes for self-guided tours, or sign language interpreters for the hearing impaired. A recent policy stipulates that all new films or videos must be captioned for the hearing impaired. The Office of Special Programs and Populations can provide contact information for individual parks. You can contact them at:

> Office of Special Programs and Populations
> National Park Service/U.S. Department of the Interior
> 800 N. Capitol NW
> Washington, DC 20002
> 202/343-3674

Planning the Amusement Park Trip

by John A. Nesbitt, Special Recreation, Inc.

1. You should contact the amusement or theme park well in advance of your trip, informing the park of the number of participants in your group and your special needs. Be sure to get in touch with person(s) responsible for special services.
2. Announce the trip well in advance and conduct a program on the trip using information available from a travel agent, the amusement park, etc.
3. Arrange your agency/institutional clearances, transportation, volunteers, food services, medical staff, etc.
4. Get all permissions (parents, family, physicians, etc.) and special instructions.
5. Screen all applicants to ensure that the trip is appropriate for each.
6. Make sure that there are suitable accommodations and services en route, at site, etc.
7. Conduct a program following the trip. Invite participants to show memorabilia or slides and photographs of the trip.

Thirteen Parks and Attractions

Several of the most beautiful national parks, along with theme parks and other tourist attractions, are listed below with accessibility information. To plan your visit or to obtain further information, you should contact the parks and attractions directly.

1. ACCESSIBLE TRAILS AT GRAND CANYON NATIONAL PARK

The terrain overall is rugged with narrow, rocky trails and steep cliffs so that visitors using wheelchairs or who are visually impaired often need assistance. The Grand Canyon National Park has brought several of its facilities up to code and has several accessible trails, lookouts, campsites and tours.

Many ranger-led programs are accessible by wheelchair and are so indicated in the park newspaper, *The Guide*.

There are accessible lodges, theaters, campgrounds, and trails. At the **North Rim** the Grand Canyon Lodge includes ramps, wheelchair lifts, cabins, restrooms, drinking fountains, snack bar, saloon. The Campground has two accessible sites.

Write to the Grand Canyon National Park and request their Accessibility Guide:

Grand Canyon National Park
P.O. Box 129
Grand Canyon, AZ 86023

2. PLAN TO VISIT SEA WORLD IN CALIFORNIA

The entire facility is accessible. This includes the Sky Ride and Sky Tower, as well as the motion-based theater. One thing to watch for—at "Mission: Bermuda Triangle" (the motion-based theater), the entire cabin moves so you need to be able to get from your wheelchair into the seats. This is true also for the Sky Ride and Sky Tower. Ramps and special seating are available for all shows. All restaurants and bathrooms are standard and have reasonable accessibility.

For further information write to:
Sea World/Guest Services
1720 South Shores Road
San Diego, CA 92109

3. WALT DISNEY WORLD—THE ACCESSIBLE MAGIC KINGDOM

Accessibility: Walt Disney World has many accessible attractions falling into three categories: 1) attractions where guests may remain in their wheelchairs throughout the attraction; 2) attractions which can accommodate guests who are able to transfer from their wheelchairs to the ride (some attractions are partially accessible to guests while in wheelchairs); 3) attractions where guests using Electric Convenience Vehicles (ECVs) must transfer to an available wheelchair or a ride vehicle to experience the attraction. Service animals are welcome in most locations throughout the Magic Kingdom, Epcot, and the Disney-MGM Studios.

Hearing Impairments: At Epcot, audio is amplified through assistive listening devices at attractions at Future World and World Showcase as well as the Disney-MGM Studios. TDDs are available at City Hall at Magic Kingdom and at Epcot locations. Guided tours of each Theme Park with Sign Language interpreters are available, with no additional charges.

Sight Impairments: Cassette tapes of pre-recorded tours are available. Relief maps of the Magic Kingdom which feature a Braille directory are posted at the Magic Kingdom at the Main Entrance and at Main Street U.S.A. Guidebooks are also available in Braille.

A detailed "Guidebook for Guests with Disabilities" is available from:

Walt Disney World
P.O. Box 10,000
Lake Buena Vista, FL 32830-1000.

4. MAMMOTH CAVE NATIONAL PARK—THE MOST FAMOUS CAVE IN AMERICA

Ranger Led Tour: Mobility Impaired Tour: 1-1/2 hrs, 1/2 mile. Designed for physically impaired visitors unable to participate in other cave tours. Ride a van to the cave and entrance and enter the cave via an elevator. See tubular passageways and delicate gypsum minerals on cave wall. Two wheelchairs are available for visitors who have not brought their own. Restrooms are not wheelchair accessible.

Heritage Trail: Near the Park Visitor Center and Hotel, the Heritage Trail offers all visitors a leisurely stroll and has been specially designed to accommodate visitors with disabilities. The trail features wheelchair turnouts, rest areas with benches, and lights for evening use. Along this trail is a beautiful overlook, large trees, and the Old Guide's Cemetery.

Headquarters Campground and Hotel: Located 1/4 mile from the Park Visitor Center, the campground has two accessible sites. The Mammoth Cave Hotel has accessible rooms. Call 502/758-2301 for details.

Mammoth Cave National Park
Mammoth Cave, KY 42259

5. THE EXTRAORDINARY SAN DIEGO ZOO AND WILD ANIMAL PARK

Hearing Impairments: Bus tours can be translated into American Sign Language with five days advance notice.

Mobility Impairment: Each bus has room for two regular sized wheelchairs or one electronic wheelchair. The Skyfari is also wheelchair accessible.

There are two moving sidewalks for access up from the lower canyon. One goes to the top of the Rain Forest Aviary, and the other goes up to Horn and Hoof Mesa.

Use of Guide and Service Dogs is heavily controlled for reasons of animal safety, but can be accommodated. It is also possible for the dog to remain in an on-site kennel free of charge while the zoo provides the visitor with an attendant to guide the park or zoo visit.

At the Wild Animal Park, the monorail tour is accessible. There is a self-guided tour booklet for the hearing impaired.

The Zoological Society of San Diego
P.O. Box 551
San Diego, CA 92112-0551
619/231-1515

6. CHICKAMAUGA AND CHATTANOOGA NATIONAL MILITARY PARK

Between 1890 and 1899 the U.S. Congress authorized the establishment of the first four military parks: Chickamauga and Chattanooga, Shiloh, Gettysburg, and Vicksburg. The first and largest of these and the one upon which the establishment and development of most of the other national military and historical parks was based was Chickamauga and Chattanooga.

Most of the facilities are accessible:

- Visitors Centers and restrooms at both Chickamauga Battlefield and Point Park on Lookout Mountain;
- The multi-media theater at Chickamauga Battlefield Visitor Ctr.;

- Wilder's Brigade Monument (tower) on Chickamauga Battlefield is accessible through a video of its interior and panoramic view from the top;
- Stops on self-guided tours at both locations;
- Three picnic areas on Chickamauga Battlefield (without restrooms) and Sanders Road picnic area (without restrooms) on Lookout Mountain;
- James Walker's 13' by 33' oil painting "The Battle Above the Clouds" with audio interpretation, located at Pt. Park Visitor Center;
- Och's Museum on the side of Lookout Mt. through a video shown on request at Point Park Visitor Center;
- Cravens House first floor is accessible and the tour of the second floor is available through a video shown on request on the first floor.

7. ACADIA NATIONAL PARK—ON THE ATLANTIC COAST

While little of New England's rockbound coast remains in public ownership, undeveloped and natural, Acadia National Park preserves the natural beauty of part of Maine's coast, its coastal mountains, and off-shore islands.

At the Park, several of the services are accessible and some are "usable" although not meeting all standards. The Thompson Island Information Center is accessible, while the Visitor and Nature Centers are usable. The Great Harbor Museum and Mt. Desert Oceanarium are also usable. Picnic and beach areas have usable sites. Campsites in the Blackwoods are accessible with paved walkways and in-car registration.

Ranger Led activities are offered mid-May to mid-October. Accessible programs will be indicated in the *Acadia Beaver Log*, the park newspaper.

Boat Cruises: Frenchman Bay Cruise is accessible. For the other cruises, deboarding may be difficult.

The park publishes the *Acadia National Park Access Guide*. You may write to:

Division of Interpretation
Acadia National Park
P.O. Box 177
Bar Harbor, ME 04069
207/288-3338

8. GULF ISLANDS NATIONAL SEASHORE—THE BARRIER ISLANDS

In the Northeastern Gulf of Mexico, Congress has set aside a few of the barrier islands for recreation and for their natural and historical resources. The park stretches from West Ship Island in Mississippi (150 miles) east to the far end of Santa Rosa Island in Florida.

The Mississippi Section: The Davis Bayou Campground has 51 sites, most with electricity and all with water hookups. The restrooms are accessible. Programs at the visitor center and fishing pier are accessible. The trip to West Ship Island is considered difficult but rewarding. The heat is intense from May-September. The boat crew will assist visitors in wheelchairs.

The Florida Section: The Visitor Centers are all accessible, as is the Museum and Auditorium. Picnic areas are accessible. Fort Pickens Campground has one accessible restroom with showers. While there are no designated accessible sites, most sites near the Loop E restroom are level. The sites have concrete pads and grass. The grills, electricity and water hookups, and picnic tables are standard. The Registration Office is not accessible.

For additional information write or call:
Gulf Islands National Seashore
1901 Gulf Breeze Parkway
Gulf Breeze, FL 32561
904/934-2600, **or**
3500 Park Rd.
Ocean Springs, MS 39564
601/875-9057

9. DENALI NATIONAL PARK AND PRESERVE—THE ALASKA REFUGE

"Denali" means the "High One" in the language of Athabascan natives and refers to the massive peak that crowns the 600-mile long Alaska Range. This is also the name of the immense national park and wildlife refuge—larger than the state of Massachusetts. The refuge contains the most varied and impressive range of wildlife on the continent. Congress designated much of Denali National Park a wilderness area which is to remain a primitive area in many respects. For the physically challenged visitor, some facilities are accessible while many are not.

The Visitor Access Center is fully accessible.

Travel on the park road is mainly done through a shuttle bus system. The number of vehicles on the roads is restricted to cause less stress to the wildlife. A bus with a wheelchair lift and extra wheelchair for loan is available with one day's notice. Special road travel passes for the severely disabled are available to those physically unable to take a bus. The Denali National Park Hotel has one room that meets current accessibility standards. Riley Creek, Savage, Teklankia and Wonder Lake have accessible campsites.

The Park has a listing of areas of the park and activities that are accessible.

For further information call 907/683-2294.

10. MESA VERDE NATIONAL PARK—THE ANCIENT CLIFFS

Mesa Verde was the home of the Anasazi Indians. They are known for their cliff dwellings It is the only national park dedicated to the works of prehistoric peoples. It consists of more than 4,000 ruin sites including 600 cliff dwellings. Elevations range from 6,500 to 8,500 feet. Spruce Tree Ruin is accessible. Most facilities have ramps. There are 6 accessible campsites.

For more information on Mesa Verde facilities, write to:

ARA Mesa Verde

P.O. Box 277

Mancos, CO 81328 (An authorized concessioner of the National Park Service)

11. EVERGLADES NATIONAL PARK—THE ENDANGERED ECOSYSTEM

The ecosystem, animal and plant life, are among the most fascinating in the United States. Known for alligators and crocodiles, for storks and hundreds of other types of birds, and for exotic waterways, the Everglades itself is severely threatened. It is one of the most popular travel spots in the U.S.

Each campground has one site reserved for visitors with disabilities. Pearl Bay Chickee, a back-country site, is accessible.

For further information, write to:

Everglades National Park

P.O. Box 279

Homestead, FL 33030

12. UNIVERSAL STUDIOS HOLLYWOOD—THE WORLD'S LARGEST STUDIO

Universal Studios has many entertainment centers and sets accessible. Only a few attractions are not accessible. Reserved seating can be arranged in advance,

The following live action shows are accessible:
· Animal Actor's Stage
· Miami Vice Action Spectacular
· The Adventures of Conan
· The Wild, Wild, Wild West Stunt Show
· The Star Trek Adventure
· An American Tail Show
· Beetlejuice's Graveyard Revue
· The Rocky and Bullwinkle Show

The tram ride is accessible and a summary is published for the hearing impaired.

For the Guide for Guests with Disabilities, please call 818/508-9600; 818/752-8514(TDD) or write to

Universal Studios HOLLYWOOD
P.O. Box 8620
Universal City, CA 91608

13. ACCESS ROCKY! VISIT THE ROCKY MOUNTAIN NATIONAL PARK

There are many accessible trails in the Rocky Mountain National Park. These trails are referred to as "universal" and represent the new art of trail design.

For the guide to accessibility at the park, write:

Rocky Mountain National Park
Estes Park, CO 80517

See, as well, an article in the Denver Post, July 4, 1995 called "Barrier-free Trails Open Up the Outdoors" by Maureen Kelly for specific trail information.

Visiting Ski Areas with Adapted Programs

Note: This information is provided by Disabled Sports, USA

Eaglecrest
Juneau, AK 99801
907/586-5284

Alpine Meadows
Tahoe City, CA 95730
916/583-4232

Alyeska Resort
(Thru Challenge Alaska)
Girdwood, AK 99587
907/783-2925

Badger Pass Ski Area
Yosemite, CA 95389
209/372-1330

Mammoth Mountain Ski Area
Mammoth, CA 93546
619/934-2571

Mt. Reba/Bear Valley
Bear Valley, CA 95223
209/753-2301

Snow Summit
Big Bear Lake, CA 92315
715/866-5766

Diamond Peak at Ski Incline
Incline Village, NV 89450
702/832-1177

Breckenridge Ski Area
Breckenridge, CO 80424
303/453-2368

Crested Butte Mountain Resort
Crested Butte, CO 81225
303/349-2333

Keystone Resort/Keystone Mountain
Keystone, CO 80435
303/468-2316
(If pre-arranged)

Powderhorn Ski Area
Mesa, CO 81643
303/242-5637

Snowmass at Aspen
Aspen, CO 81615
303/923-1220
800/525-6200

Steamboat Ski Area
Steamboat Springs, CO 80487
303/879-6111
(By appointment)

Vail
Vail, CO 81658
303/476-5601
(By appointment)

Winter Park Resort
Winter Park, CO 80482
303/726-5514

Santa Fe Ski Area
Santa Fe, NM 87501
505/982-4429

Ski Apache
(Thru: Ski Apache Handicapped
Association)
Ruidoso, NM 88345
505/336-4356

Mt. Bachelor
Bend, OR 97709
503/382-2607 (Mountain)
503/382-2442 (Corp. Office)

Park City Ski Area
Park City, UT 84060
801/649-8111 (Pre-arranged)

**Snowbird Ski and Summer
Resort**
Snowbird, UT 84092
801/742-2222 (Pre-arranged)

**Alpental/Snoqualmie (Ski
Areas)**
Snoqualmie Pass
Snoqualmie, WA 98068
206/434-6112 (Alpental; 6671
S.A.)
206/434-6161 (Snoqualmie)

Crystal Mountain
Crystal Mountain, WA 98022
206/663-2265
(Lessons, rates and services upon
reservation)

Hyland Hills Ski Area
Bloomington, MN 55438
612/835-4745

Spirit Mountain Rec. Area
Duluth, MN 55810
218/628-2891

Welch Village
Welch, MN 55089

612/222-7079
612/222-9145 or
612/258-4567

Wisp Ski Area
McHenry, MD 21541
301/387-4911

The Homestead Ski Area
Hot Springs, VA 24445
703/839-7721

Massanutten
Harrisonburg, VA 22801
703/289-9441

Canaan Valley Resort
Davis, WV 26260
304/866-4121

Wachusett Mountain
Princeton, MA 01541
508/464-5101

Bristol Mountain
Canandaigua, NY 14424
716/374-6331

Gore Mountain Ski Area
North Creek, NY 12853
518/251-2411

Hunt Hollow Ski Club
Naples, NY 14512
716/374-5428

Kissing Bridge
Glenwood, NY 14069
716/592-4963

Hunter Mountain Ski Bowl
Hunte, NY 12442
518/263-4223

Ski Windham
Windham, NY 12496
518/734-4300

Bromley Mountain
Manchester Center, VT 05152
802/824-5522

Jack Frost
Blakesley, PA 18610
717/443-8425, ext. 351

Whitetail
Mercersburg, PA
717/328-9400
(call to arrange)

CANADA

Marmot Basin
Jasper, Alberta TOE lEO
403/852-3816

Sunshine Village
Banff, Alberta TOL OCO
403/762-6500

Fernie Snow Valley
Fernie, BC VOB lBO
604/423-4655

Whistler/Blackcomb Mountains
Whistler, BC VON 1BO
604/932-3434 (Whistler)
604/932-3141 (Blackcomb)

Ski Martock
Windsor, Nova Scotia Bon 2TO
902/798-9501

Calabogie Peaks
Calabogie, Ontario
613/752-2720

Chedoke Winter Sports PK
Hamilton, Ontario
416/528-0355

Horseshoe Valley Resort
Horseshoe Valley, Ontario
705/835-3790
416/283-2988

Le Valinouet
Falandean, Quebec
418/696-1962

Mont-Sainte-Anne (Par du)
Beaupre; Quebec GOA lEO
418/827-4561

Wheelchair Basketball

Wheelchair basketball is the most popular and widely known of the wheelchair sports. The National Wheelchair Basketball Association is the national governing body for wheelchair basketball; as such it promotes and governs the sport and sanctions tournaments and events. The following list includes the NWBA's women's division, youth division, independents, conferences, and conference members. From this roster you should be able to locate the teams nearest you.

WOMEN'S DIVISION

Chairperson
Sharon Hedrick
2808 Susan Stone Drive
Urbana, IL 61801
(217) 337-3490 (W)

Vice Chairperson
Deb Sunderman
13629 Glendale Trail
Savage, MN 55378
(612) 447-4139 (W)
(612) 894-6238 (H)

Secretary
Pat Ninke
1073 W. 13th St. #4
San Pedro, CA 90731
(310) 548-1927 (H)

Bay Area Meteorites
Kathryn Black
4130 Webster St. #2
Oakland, CA 94609
(510) 849-4663 (W)

Texas Heat
Pam Fontaine
1510 Woodcreek Dr.
Richardson, TX 75082
(214) 907-9468

Minnesota Women's Timber-wolves
Perry Hendricks
5904 Cahill Ave. E.
Inver Grove Hgts, MN 55076
(612) 455-7907
(Tel/Fax)

Continental Community Team
Rob McCarthy
P.O. Box 567
Chandler, AZ 85244
(602) 917-2195

RIC Express
RIC-Wirtz Sports Program
345 E. Superior
Chicago, IL 60611
(312) 908-4292 (W)
Fax (312) 908-1051

Irvine Valley College Lasers
Mikel Bistany
550 Irvine Center Dr.
Irvine, CA 92720
(714) 559-3243 (W)
(714) 646-3669 (H)

Univ. of Illinois Fighting Illini
Brad Hedrick
136 Rehab Educ. Center
University of Illinois

1207 S. Oak Street
Champaign, IL 61820
(217) 333-4606 (W)

Southern California Sunrise
Pat Ninke
(see Secretary, above)

YOUTH DIVISION

President
Barb Radbel
9149 Marigold Lane
Munster, IN 46321
(219) 838-8562

Vice President
Bob Trotter
60 E. 36th Place #604
Chicago, IL 60653
(312) 268-5144 (H)
(708) 687-7200x3530

Secretary
Karsten Vollstedt
500 East Roosevelt
Appleton, WI 54911
(414) 733-3381 (H)
(414) 731-2435
(414) 731-3278 (W)

Treasurer
Tom Becke
109 West State Rd #231
Crown Point, IN
(219) 663-5260 (H)
(312) 767-3300 (W)
(312) 767-9652 Fax

Commissioner
Robert J. Szyman
St. Louis Wheelchair Athletic
Association
6420 Clayton Road

St. Louis, MO 63117
(314) 768-5325 (W)
Fax (314) 768-5316

BORP Bay Cruisers
Tim Orr/Kathryn Black
BORP
830 Bancroft Way
Berkeley, CA 94710
(510) 849-4663 (W)
(415) 824-3938 (H)
(510) 849-4616 Fax

Courage Youth Sports
C. J. Maichen Courage Center
3915 Golden Valley Road
Golden Valley, MN 55422
(612) 520-0482 (W)
(612) 992-8813 (H)
(612) 520-0577 Fax

Dallas Junior Texans
Stephanie Reeves
600 Sherwood Court
Irving, TX 75061
(214) 423-4482

Spalding Spartans
Walt Coffey
Spalding School
1628 West Washington
Chicago, IL 60612
(312) 534-7438

CAWS Rolling Rebels —Indiana
Barb Radbel
9149 Marigold Lane
Munster, IN 46321
(219) 838-8562

Kentwood Junior Pacers
Theresa Rettig
Kentwood Recreation Dept.
355 48th St., SE
Kentwood, MI 49548

(616) 531-2391
(616) 531-3820 Fax

Kansas City Junior Pioneers
Mike Morrissey
P.O. Box 3569
Kansas City, KS 66103
(913) 492-8136 (W)

Los Angeles Kodiaks
Les Hayes
Widney High School
2302 South Gramercy Place
Los Angeles, CA 90018
(310)731-8633

Mad City Junior Bombers
Jean Winters
1045 East Dayton St. #103
Madison, WI 53703
(608) 271-1572 (H)
(608) 266-6454 (W)

Manitoba Junior Team
Manitoba Wheelchair Sports
200 Main Street
Winnipeg, Manitoba R3C 4M2

Sioux Junior Wheelers
David Van Buskirk
616 North Nesmith
Sioux Falls, SD 57103-0844
(605) 334-0000 (H)
(605) 366-0202 (W)

St. Louis Rolling Rams
Robert J. Szyman
(see Commissioner, above)

Tulsa Jammers
Ken Lee
Center for the Physically Limited
815 S. Utica Avenue
Tulsa, OK 74104
(918) 584-8607 (W)
(918) 437-1412 (H)
(918) 584-8646 Fax

CAWS — Illinois
Sue Dineen
7326 North Oketo
Chicago, IL 60631
(312) 774-3676 (H)
(312) 534-7436 (W)

Variety Village
Stephen Bialows
Variety Village
3701 Danforth Avenue
Scarborough, Ontario MlN 2G2
(416) 699-7167

Wisconsin Junior Horizons
Karsten Volstedt
500 East Roosevelt
Appleton, WI 54911
(414) 733-3381 (H)
(414) 731-2435
(414) 731-3278 (W)

**Arkansas Junior Rolling'
Razorbacks**
Doug Garner
122 Mesa Trail
Hot Springs, AR 71813
(501) 767-9185 (H)
(501) 525-4503 (W)

Massachusetts Chariots
Theorize Kelly
3 Randolf Street
Canton, MA 02021
(617) 878-2440x386 (W)
(617) 821-4086 Fax
(617) 863-1780 (H)

Nebraska
Karin Johnson
Benson Community Center
6008 Maple Street
Omaha, NE 68104
(402) 444-5184 (W)

Chicago Wheelchair Bulls
NEDSRA
Attn. Craig Culp
1770 W. Centennial Place
Addison, Illinois 60101
(708) 620-4500 (W)
(708) 620-4598 Fax

North Carolina Wheels of Steel
John Ferguson
502 Applecross
Cary, NC 27511
(919) 460-5975

Twin City Spinners Jrs.
Karen Walsh
124 Moccasin Drive
Waterloo, Ontario
Canada N2L 4C3
(519) 741-1756 (W)
(519) 747-5714 (H)
(519) 741-9771 FAX

**NWBA INDEPENDENTS
(Non-Conference Affiliated)**

Buffalo EPVA Chariots
Mark J. Dunford
111 W. Huron Street
Buffalo, NY 14202
(716) 846-4532 (W)

Dallas Mavericks
Abu Yilla
970 Duncan Perry #1032
Grand Prairie, TX 75050
(817) 898-2575 (W)
(214) 602-0833 (H)

Golden State Warriors
Bill Duncan
870 Hilmar Street
Santa Clara, CA 95050

(415) 361-3814 (W)
(408) 241-1877 (H)

Cleveland Wheelchair Cavs
Lynn Charles
Cleveland Cavs
1 Center Court
Cleveland, OH 44115
(216) 420-2227 (W)
(216) 420-2101 FAX
(216) 464-2866 (H)

Dallas Texans
Sam Seidemann
Rt. 1, Box 171
Nevada, TX 75173
(214) 843-2455

Fresno Red Rollers
Wayne Kunishige
7289 N. Brooks
Fresno, CA 93711
(209) 292-2171 (W)
(209) 438-0908 (H)
(209) 292-2741 FAX

London Forest City Flyers
Paul Bowes
72 Knightsbridge Road
London, Ontario N6K 3R4
Canada
(519) 681-1441 (W)
(519) 471-4189 (H)
(519) 642-3446 FAX

Rochester Wheels
Stephen Barbados
41 Cave Hollow
W. Henrietta, NY 14586
(716) 275-3483 (W)
(716) 256-0423 FAX
(716) 359-0818 (H)

Ottawa Royals
Reg McClelland
1600 James Naismith Dr.

Gloucester, Ont. K1B 5N4
Canada
(613) 748-5888 (W)
(613) 837-1824 (H)
(613) 748-5889 FAX

Temple Univ. Rollin' Owls
Tribit Green
Recreation Services
1858 N. Broad Street
Temple University
Philadelphia, PA 19121
(215) 204-4783 (W)
(215) 849-9487 (H)

Univ. of Arizona Wildchairs
Dave Herr-Cardillo
Center for Disability Related
Resources
University of Arizona
Tucson, AZ 85721
(602) 622-1752 (H)
(602) 621-5178 (W)
FAX (602) 621-9423

Twin City Spinners
Bruce Russell
520 Mortimer Drive
Cambridge, Ont. N3H 5M5
(519) 621-2130x2818 (W)
(519) 650-3903 (H)
(519) 623-8234 FAX

Phoenix Outlaws
Tammy Townsend
1625 E. Cambridge #1
Phoenix, AZ 85006
(602) 241-1484

Northcoast Action (OH)
David Williams
901 Shadylawn
Amherst, OH 44001-1747
(216) 329-6989 (W)
(Z16) 985-2038 (H)
(216) 366-9008 FAX

Orlando Magic Wheels
Roger Davis
307 Double Springs Rd.
Murfreesboro, TN 37130
(615) 862-4925
(615) 895 -8861 (H)
(615) 862-4429 FAX

Utah Wheelin' Jazz
Mike Schlappi
2042 E. Windsor Oak Cove
Sandy, UT 84092
(801) 572-1350 (H)
(800) 944-4750 (W)
FAX (801) 532-3098

Manasota (FL) Hurricanes
Richard Montgomery
1840 2nd Ave. East
Bradenton, FL 34208
(813) 497-6388 (W)
(813) 746-9078 (H)

Rochester Wheels
Stephen Barbados
41 Cave Hollow
W. Henrietta, NY 14586
(716) 275-3483 (W)
(716) 256-0423 FAX
(716) 359-0818 (H)

ARKANSAS VALLEY

President
Mike Childers
8439 East 24 Street
Tulsa, OK 74129-2903
(918) 663-1940 (H)

Vice President
Mike Baker
8370 E. 16 St. So.
Muskogee, OK 74403

(918) 682-3364 (W)
(918) 683-5427 (H)

Secretary
Pat Childers (see Mike, above)

Treasurer
Doug Moore
905 Anderson Way
Van Buren, AR 72956
(501) 471-4314 (W)
(501) 474-0825 (H)

Commissioner
Harry Vines
2005 Broken Bow
No. Little Rock, AR 72116
(800) 622-4472 (W)
(501) 682-2642 (W)
(501) 834-8513 (H)

Ft. Smith
Doug Moore (see Treasurer, above)

Okie Spokesmen
Jon Bostic
Box 75554
Okla City, OK 73147
(405) 945-4499 (W)
 (405) 521-0628 (H)

Muskogee Rollin' Raiders
John Benson
7450 W. 43 St. So.
Muskogee, OK 74401
(918) 687-0167 (H)

Tulsa Rollin' Roustabouts
Bill Smith
8439 East 24 Street
Tulsa, OK 74129
(918) 663-1940 (H)

Conf. Independent

Arkansas Rollin' Razorbacks
Cheryl Vines
2005 Broken Bow
No. Little Rock, AR 72116
(501) 324-9624 (W)
(501) 834-8513 (H)
(501) 296-1787 FAX

CAPITAL

President
Mickey Toombs
906 Bonita Road
Richmond, VA 23227
(804) 262-1850 (H)
(804) 367-0954 (W)

Vice President
Jim Leatherman 4019 Putty Hill
Avenue Baltimore, MD 21236
(410) 668-5787 (H) (410)
965-1141 (W)

Secretary/ Treasurer
Nancy Leatherman
4019 Putty Hill Avenue
Baltimore, MD 21236
(410) 668-5787 (H)

Commissioner
Cecil W. Wood
P.O. Box 735
Edgewood, MD 21040
(410) 569-3810 (H)

Charlotte Cardinals
Herman Key
201 W. Main, #8
Charlottesville, CA 22902
(804) 293-6843 (H)
(804) 971-9629 (W)

Hampton/Newport News Peninsula Magic
Stephanie Crump
22 Lincoln Street
Hampton, VA 23669
(804) 727-1601 (W)
(804) 596-8150 (H)

Richmond Rimriders
Jim May
2641 Sandhurst Lane
Midlothian, VA 23113
(804) 794-7447

NRH Ambassadors
Taimi Paadre
Community Relations
102 Irving St. NW
Washington, DC 20010
(202) 877-1779 (W)
(301) 989-9383 (H)

Virginia Beach Sun Wheelers
St. Clair Jones, Jr.
2289 Lynnhaven Pkwy.
Virginia Beach, VA 23456
(804) 421-2891 (H)
(804) 471-5884 (W)

CAROLINAS

President
Jeff Brafford
14101 Fountain Lane
Charlotte, NC 28278
(704) 376-5555 (W)
(7()4) 588-2133 (H)

Vice President
Ted Williamson
2755 New Blockhouse
Maryville, TN 37801
(615) 983-9182 (H)

Secretary
Randy Ward
Rt. 5, Box 40
Whiteville, NC 28472
(910) 642-8617 (H)

Treasurer
Bruce Hankins
Rt. 3, Box 638
Ridgeway, VA 24148
(703) 956-2881 (H)
(703) 632-2062x366 (W)

Commissioner
Ken Fullbright
26 Lake Shore Dr.
Weaverville, NC 28787
(704) 255-7710 (W)
(704) 658-2315 (H)

Division I

East Tennessee Wheelbillies
Ted Williamson
(see VP, above)

Charlotte Hornets
Jeff Brafford
(see President, above)

Roanoke Star City Saints
Bruce Hankins
(see Treasurer, above)

Carolina Tarwheels
Dick Bryant
8245 Charles Crawford Lane
Charlotte, NC 28262
(704) 547-0176 (H)

Division II

Wake Wheelers
Terrence Smith
85 Montgomery Heights Rd.
Selma, NC 27576
(919) 965-5254

Augusta Rack-n-Rollers
David McNeil
102 Wesley Drive
Martinez, GA 30907
(706) 860-1012 (W)
(706) 863 -2496 (H)

Carolina Express
Randy Ward
(see Secretary, above

Port City Spokesmen
Chris Doody
747 Timber Lane
Wilmington, NC 28405
(910) 452-1434

CENTRAL INTERCOLLE-GIATE

President
Jim Hayes
Box 19348 UTA Station
Arlington, TX 76019
(817) 273-3364
FAX (817) 273-2962

Vice President
Brad Hedrick
University of Illinois
Rehab-Educ. Center
1207 Oak Street
Champaign, IL 61820
(217) 333-4606
FAX (217) 333-0248

Secretary/Treasurer
Lew Shaver
CA 122
Southwest State University
Marshall, MN 56258
(507) 537-6298
FAX (507) 537-7154

Commissioner
Dan Byrnes
Recreation Programs
203 lrving Gymnasium
Ball State University
Muncie, IN 47306
(317) 285-1753 (W)
FAX (317) 285-5353

UTA Movin' Mavs
Jim Hayes
(see President, above)

Univ. of Wis./Whitewater War-hawks
Mike Frogley Disabled Student Services 1004 Roseman Univ. Wisc./Whitewater Whitewater, WI 53190 (414) 472-3169 (W) FAX (414) 472-5210

Southwest St. Univ.
Lew Shaver
(see Sec./Treas., above)

Univ. of Illinois Fighting Illini
Brad Hedrick
(see VP, above)

Southern IL Univ.
Kim Martin
Southern Illinois Univ.
Campus Recreation
Carbondale, IL 62901
(618) 536-5531
FAX (618) 453-1238

EASTERN

President
Ed Waluk
256 Barton Ave.
Patchogue, NY 11772
(718) 990-7819 (W)

(516) 654-5130 (H)
FAX (718) 526-0987

Vice President
Charles Gray
109-13 157th Street
Jamaica, NY 11433
(718) 529-7364 (H)

Secretary
Pete Cimino
3199 Eastern Parkway
Baldwin, NY 11510
(516) 223-8087 (H)
(516) 572-0251 (W)

Treasurer
Sylvester Simmons
225 East 93rd St. #8a
New York, NY 10128
(212) 996-3929 (H)
(718) 424-2929x23 (W)
FAX (718) 335-0545

Commissioner
Joseph Luceri
444 East 20th Street, #3a
New York, NY 10009
(212) 456-3351 (Nights)
(212) 979-7530 (H)
FAX (212) 456-3399

Brooklyn Whirlaways
David White
56 7th Ave. #1OJ
New York, NY 10011
(212) 691-1975 (H)

Nassau Kings
Tony Fitzgerald
257 Covert Ave.
Floral Park Crest,
NY 11 001
(516) 488-6248 (H)

Woodside Blazers
Sylvester Simmons

(see Treasurer, above)

EPVA Chargers
Al Youakim
174 Ruckman Rd.
Hillsdale, NJ 07642
(201) 664-6882 (H)

Long Island Express
Angelo Cardinale
155 Huron St.
Howard Beach, NY 11414
(713) 835-9763 (H)

KEYSTONE

President
Darius Carlins
3147 Churchview Avenue
Pittsburgh, PA 15227
(412) 884-5784 (H)

Vice President
Tim Gorby
1309 Lowe Elkton
Columbiana, OH 44408
(216) 482-3451

Secretary
Bob Shomo
848 Lucas Place
Johnstown, PA 15901
(814) 734-4720 (H)
(814) 732-2462 (W)

Treasurer
Mike Auer
101 N. Mill, Apt. 110
Ridgway, PA 15853
(814) 772-9166 (H)

Commissioner
John Sikora
118 Sunset Drive
Sarver, PA 16055

Sports, Everyone!

(412) 295-5263 (H)
(412) 826-2771 (W)
(412) 828-0748 FAX

Akron Rubber City Rollers
Alan Burgess
3687 Hiwood Avenue
Stow, OH 44224
(216) 688-0126 (H)
(216) 653-7755 (W)

Edinboro University Rolling Scots
Robin Boyd
ODSS, Shafer Hall
Edinboro U. of PA
Edinboro, PA 16444
(814) 732-2462 (W)

Carbon City Rollers
Bob Mecca/Mike Auer
Comm. Res. for Ind.
503 Arch Street
St. Mary's, PA 15857
(814) 781-3050 (W)
(814) 781-1635 (H)

Pittsburgh Steelwheelers
Darius Carlins
(see President, above)

Youngstown YMCA Hot Wheels
Rick Greenfield
2918 1/2 Roosevelt
Youngstown, OH 44504
(800) 777-1691 (W)
(216) 759-3002 (H)

Johnstown Flood City Wheelers
Doug Neal
R.D. #1, Box 85
Smicksburg, PA 16256
(412) 286-3286 (H)

LAKE MICHIGAN

President/Secretary
Jim Taylor
1007 Swain
Elmhurst, IL 60126
(708) 832-2914 (H)
(312)686-6173 (W)

Vice President
John Beck
1040 N. 2nd St.
c/o Ramp, Inc.
Rockford, IL 61107
(815) 397-2720 (H)
(815) 968-7467 (W)

Treasurer
Bob Kroon
221 Edison Park, NW
Grand Rapids, MI 49504
(616) 453-5619 (H)

Commissioner
Tom Cunningham
4632 N. Winchester
Chicago, IL 60640
(312) 334-5864

Rockford Chariots
John Beck
(see VP, above)

Quint-Cities Roughriders
Joe Daebelliehn
1102 25th St.
Moline, IL 61265
(309) 788-6117 (W)
(309) 764-5803 (H)

RIC Hornets
Tom Richey
Rehabilitation
Institute of Chicago
345 E. Superior

Chicago, IL 60611
(312) 908-4292 (W)

Conference Independents

Grand Rapids Pacers
Bob Groggel
22916 66th Ave.
Mattawan, MI 49071
(616) 668-4731 (H)
(616) 341-6325 (W)

Chicago Bulls
Jim Taylor
(see President, above)

LONE STAR

President
Michael J. Barr
3515 Hideaway Lane
Spring, TX 77388
(713) 350-6029

Vice President
Buddy Johnson
Rt. 1, Box 318-H
Winnie, TX 77665
(409) 296-9826 (W)

Secretary/Treasurer
Oran Burnett
11951 Dawn Haven
San Antonio,TX 78249
(210) 826-7727 (H)

Commissioner
Tom Brown
VA Hospital (llK)
7400 Merton Minter Blvd.
San Antonio, TX 78284
(210) 617-5125 (W)

Beaumont
Buddy Johnson (see VP, above)

Austin Rec'ers
Bryson McCall Smith
4210 Red River #123
Austin, TX 78751
(512) 453-1014

Houston Rolling Cougars
Johnny Banda
12801 Roydon #2103
Houston, TX 77034
(713) 481-3932 (H)

San Antonio Spurs
Oran Burnett
(see Secretary, above)

South Texas Chariots
Gustavo Quintero
1711 Kristi Lane
Mission, TX 78572
(512) 581-8703

Houston Rollin' Rockets
Jeff Williams
P.O. Box 154
Pattison, TX 77466
(713) 375-5130 (H)
(713) 932-7477 (W)

MID-AMERICA

President
Stephen Miller
1616 Muirridge Court
Batavia, OH 45103
(513)753-1054

Vice President
Tom Stokes
582 Hillcreek Road
Shepherdsville, KY 40165
(502) 957-5865

Treasurer
Terry DeHaai

Sports, Everyone!

P.O. Box 363
Dayton, IN 47941
(317) 296-2019

Commissioner
Joseph Gschwender, Jr.
400 Sycamore Street
Brookville, OH 45309
(513) 833-3180

Queen City Slammers (Cincinatti)
Stephen Miller
(see President, above)

Lafayette Spinners
Terry Niccum
1712 Morton Street
Lafayette, IN 47904
(317) 742-4815

Dayton Raiders
Jim Munson
15A Old Yellow Sp. Rd.
Fairborn, OH 45324
(513) 879-5045

Miami Valley Rollers (Dayton)
Gene Leber
1236 Freeman Drive
Beavercreek, OH 45434
(513) 429-8817

Indiana Wheelchair Pacers
(Indianapolis)
Jeff Ramon
512 North Denny
Indianapolis, IN 46201
(317) 356-2330

Ohio Buckeye Wheelers
(Columbus)
Rick Morrison
6355 Buckeye Path N.
Grove City, OH 43123-959
(614) 875-1683

Ann Arbor Thunderbirds
Kevin Wolf
2277 Bryn Mawr #713W
Ypsilanti, MI 48198
(313) 480-2419

Louisville Mustangs
Tom Stokes
(see VP, above)

MID-ATLANTIC

President
Joe Thieringer
13 Akron Avenue
Westmont, NJ 08108
(609) 869-0648

Vice President
Eugene Barlow
70 Federal court
Absecon, NJ 08201
(609) 652-6119 (H)

Secretary
Jayne Marie Eagle
223 Scottdale Rd. B411
Lansdowne, PA 19050
(215) 623-8953 (H)

Treasurer
Angelo Mongiovi
41 S. 20th St.
Kenilworth, NJ 07033
(908) 276-5846 (H)
(210) 898-8312 (W)
(201) 898-8116 FAX

Commissioner
Dan Sullivan
1521 Hollinshed Ave.
Pennsauken, NJ 08110
(609) 663-1338 (H)

(215) 587-3080 (W)
(215) 587-9216 FAX

New Jersey Blue Devils
Matt Darlow
45-1512 River Dr. S.
Jersey City, NJ 07310
(201) 626-3464 (H)
(201) 882-5455 (W)
FAX (201) 882-8076

Philadelphia Spokesmen
Jayne Marie Eagle
(see Secretary, above)

DMPVA Streaks
Randy McGlocklin
43 Carlisle Road
Newark, DE 19713
(302) 737-4355 (H)
(302) 739-9599 (W)
(302) 739-6285 FAX

Newark Renegades
Shelton Harding
6B Independence Cirole
Newark, DE 19711
(302) 737-9773 (H)

Jersey Shore High Rollers
John Portelli
343 Madison Ave.
Bayville, NJ 08721
(908) 269-3076 (H)
(908) 269-3528 FAX

Scranton Allied Forces
Jim Batton
Allied Services Rehab Hosp.
475 Morgan Hwy. Box 1103
Scranton, PA 18501
(717) 348-1397 (W)
(717) 348-1261 (FAX)
(717) 587-0416 (H)

MIDWEST

President
Ron Maurer
14858 Ralls Lane
Bridgeton, MO 63044
(314) 770-2475 (H)
(314) 994-2132 (W)
(314) 994-0067 FAX

Vice President
Mike Peters
4018 SW 43rd St.
Topeka, KS 66610
(913) 267-7046 (H)
(913) 296-0970 (W)

Treasurer
Randy Fisher
(see Commissioner below)

Secretary
Robert Szyman
St. Louis W.A.A.
6420 Clayton Road
St. Louis, MO 63117-1872
(314) 768-5325
(FAX) (314) 768-5316

Commissioner
Randy Fisher
7233 SW Timberway Drive
Topeka, KS 66619-1173
(913) 296-5005 (W)

Kansas City Rolling Pioneers
Dave Pierce
8422 Flora
Kansas City, MO 64131
(816)523-1249 (H)

St. Louis Rolling Rams
Julie Treadway
#11 Weinel
Fairview Hgts, IL 62208

(618) 398-5750 (H)
(314) 577-5669 (W)
(314) 577-5366 FAX

Northeast Kansas Wheelhawks
Andy Hanschu
2501 SE Michigan
Topeka, KS 66605
(913) 233-1951 (H)

University of Illinois —Fighting Illini—Men
Brad Hedrick
136 Rehab Educ. Center
University of Illinois
1207 South Oak Street
Champaign, IL 61820
(217) 333-4606 (W)

NORTH CENTRAL

President
Karen Casper-Robeson
7829 61st Ave. North
New Hope, MN 55428
(612) 520-0311 (W)
(612) 533-4769 (H)
(612) 520-0577 FAX

Vice President
Susan Hagel
Sister Kenny Institute
800 E. 28th St. at Chicago Ave.
Minneapolis, MN 55407
(612) 863-5712 (W)
(612) 546-6069 (H)
(612) 863-4507 FAX

Secretary/Treasurer
Perry Hendricks
5904 Cahill Ave. East
Inver Grove Hgts, MN 55076
455-7907 (H) and FAX

Commissioner
Jim Olson
Lutheran Brotherhood
625 Fourth Avenue South
Minneapolis, MN 55414
(612) 340-8014 (W)
(612) 479-6443 (H)
(612) 340-8389 FAX

North Dakota Wallbangers
Craig Charbonneau
1104 Oak Street
Grand Forks, ND 58201
(701) 77Z-8142

Key City Rollers
Dick Crumb
1631 Castle Drive
No. Mankato, MN 56003
(507) 389-9006 (H)
(507) 387-4174 (W)

Courage Rolling Timberwolves—Men
Tobe Broadrick
Courage Center
3915 Golden Valley Rd
Golden Valley, MN 554
(612) 520-0479 (W)
(612) 566-5755 (H)
(612) 520-0577 FAX

Courage Rolling Gophers—Men
Steve Hanson
1435 Hampshire Ave. South #107
2 St. Louis Park, MN 55426
(612) 542-9352 (H)
(612) 929-1050 (W)

Southwest State University Broncos
Lew Shaver
BA 122 SWSU

Marshall, MN 56258
(507) 532-7355 (H)
(507) 537-7271 (6298)

Sioux Wheelers
David VanBuskirk
616 N. Nesmith Ave.
Sioux Falls, SD 57103
(605) 334-0000 (H)
(605) 366-0202 (W)

Twin Port Flyers
Charlie Wittwer
4239 Birch Valley Rd.
Hermantown, MN 55811
(218) 726-4404 (W)
(218) 729-9099 (H)

Rochester Cowboys
Maynard Read
325 1st Ave. SW 106
Rochester, MN 55901
(507) 287-6193 (H)
(507) 282-8284 (W)

NORTHEAST

President
Jay Kennedy
23 Farm Drive
E. Hartford, CT 06108
(203) 289-2524 (H)
(203) 525-6758 (W)

Vice President
Scott Factor
57 Will Dr. #166
Canton, MA 02021
(617) 828-6686 (H)
(617) 740-2300 (W)

Treasurer
Bill Dombroski
249 W. Park Ave.

New Haven, CT 06511
(203) 469-3562 (H)
(203) 389-1569 (W)

Secretary
Joe Bellil
22-4 Williamsburg Ct.
Shrewsbury, MA 01545
(508) 842-2596 (H)

Commissioner
Al Youakim
174 Ruckman Road
Hillsdale, NJ 07642
(201) 664-6882 (H)

Bay State Machine
Mike Kennedy
158 N. Main St.
Millbury, MA 01527
(508) 865-2655 (H)
(800) 358-4579 (W)

Park City Rollers
Norm Message
601 Valley Road
Fairfield, CT 06432
(203) 374-8072 (H)

NEPVA Blazers
Eddie Buckley
43 Garden Street
W. Newbury, MA 01985
(508) 465-9583

Rhode Island Rhode Runners
Tom Dodd
43 Harding Road
North Kingston, RI 02852
(401) 884-6623

Connecticut Spokebenders
Tom Morrison
81 North St.
Manchester, CT 06040
(203) 645-0646 (H)

Adirondack Thunder Rolling
Adam Sheehan
1925 8th Avenue
Watervliet, NY 12189
(518) 274-6197 (H)

NEPVA Celtics
Paul Cowan
17 Bennett Dr. #3
Stoughton, MA 02072
(617) 344-1472 (H)
(508) 880-4117 (W)

NORTHWEST

President
Scott Boyles
13981 S.E. Lucille Street
Happy Valley, OR 97Z36-5606
(503) 760-6480 (H)
(503) 654-4333 (W)
(503) 654-8330 FAX

Vice President
Bob LaFavor
88618 Chukar Lane
Veneta, OR 97487
(503) 935-7770

Secretary/Treasurer
Kathie Panciarelli
2082 NW 15th Court
Gresham, OR 97030
(503) 661-1987

Conference Commissioner
Bill Donahue
1803 West Glass
Spokane, WA 99205
(509) 325-1290 (H)
(509) 456-2262 (W)

Federal Way Federals
Joseph DiBernardo
l2544 SE 72nd St.
Renton, WA 98056
(206) 228-4005

Portland Wheelblazers
Kirk Parkhurst
1437 SE Beech St.
Gresham, OR 97030
(503) 661-3248

Rip City Rollers
Carl Backstrom
3589 SE Monroe #27
Milwaukie, OR 97222
(503) 653-5315

Seattle Supersonics
Douglas Lee
5735 59th Ave. NE
Seattle, WA 98422
(206) 526-0671 (H)
(206) 821-1010 (W)

Spokane Cyclones
John Rees
S. 508 Henry Rd.
Greenacres, WA 99016
(509) 928-3102 (H)

West Plains Drifters
Walt Mabe
S. 21423 Beckley Lane
Cheney, WA 99004
(509) 235-6049 (H)

**Willamette Valley Rollin'
Rebels**
James Cook
4685 Hayesville Court, NE
Salem, OR 97305
(503) 390-2688 (H)

PACIFIC COAST

President
Leroy Ransom
3460 West 7th Street #212
Los Angeles, CA 90005
(213) 731-8633 (W)
(213) 383-2396 (H)

Secretary
Pat Ninke
1073 W. 13th St. #4
San Pedro, CA 90731
(310) 548-1927

Treasurer
Marty Todd
3129 Yearling St.
Lakewood, CA 90712
(310) 633-7540

Commissioner
Bill Johnson
814 Cartagena Street
Long Beach, CA 90807
(310) 427-6340

Widney HS Kodiaks
Les Hayes
3529 Oak Avenue
Manhattan Bch, CA 90266
(213) 731-8633 (W)
(310) 545-6790 (H)

Rancho Renegades
Lisa Hilborn
955 E. 3rd #208
Long Beach, CA 90802
(310) 495-0177
(310) 940-7201

Southern California Sunrise
Pat Ninke (see
Secretary, above)

Los Angeles Mayas
Hector Jiminez
3727 W. 6th St.
Suite 511
Los Angeles, CA 90020
(213) 732-3187 (H)
(310) 314-9873 (W)

Pasadena Big Wheels
Hector Rodriguez
430 E. Adams Blvd.
Los Angeles, CA 90011
(213) 746-7512 (H)

Conference Independent

Long Beach Flying Wheels
Mike Junghanel
3423 Volk Avenue
Long Beach, CA 90808
(714) 435-2443 (W)
(310) 429-8843 (H)

Los Angeles Stars
Oscar Sepulveda
315 Myers Place
Inglewood, CA 90301
(310) 677-5841 (H)
(310) 825-3317 (W)

ROCKY MOUNTAIN

President
Jeffrey L. Deaver
523 Ellis Court
Golden, CO 80401
(303) 288-8484 (W)
(303) 279-6491 (H)

Vice President
Cliff Coker
6559 Lewis Court
Arvada, CO 80004

Sports, Everyone!

(303) 369-1714 (W)
(303) 421-3882 (H)

Secretary
Mike Lovato
4300 David Court
Rio Rancho, MN 87124
(505) 891-0346 (H)
(505) 764-6850 (W)

Treasurer
Joe Gomez
(see Commissioner, below)

Commissioner
Joe Gomez
Craig Hospital
3425 S. Clarkson
Englewood, CO 80110
(303) 789-8313 (W)
(303) 753-0696 (H)

Colorado Rolling Cowboys
Larry Smith
8583 W. Pacific Place
Lakewood, CO 80227
(303) 989-4318 (H)

Albuquerque PVA Zia Storm
Mike Lovato
(see Secretary, above)

Colorado Springs Steam Roll-ers
Steve Mixon
4825 Astrozom Bld. 281
Colorado Springs, CO 80916
(719) 392-8310

Denver Nuggets
Jeffrey L. Deaver
(see President, above)

SOUTHERN

President
Leland Meeks
7469 Hooper Cove Road
Young Harris, GA 30582
(706) 379-1606 (H)

Vice President
Mike Neville
627 Heflin Ave. East
Birmingham, AL 35214
(205) 791-1291 (H)

Secretary/Treasurer
Butch Martin
5454 South Hilltop Drive
Mobile, AL 36608
(205) 344-2750 (H)

Commissioner
Roger Davis, Jr.
1536 Heritage View Blvd.
Madison, TN 37115
(615) 865-8958 (H)
(615) 862-4894 (W)

East Division

Lakeshore Pioneers
Frank T. Burns
3800 Ridgeway Dr.
Birmingham, AL 35209
(205) 871-0367 (H)
(205) 868-2310 (W)

Lakeshore Chariots
Frank T. Burns (see Pioneers)

Nashville Wheelcats
Mike Sells
717 Honey Grove Ct.
Antioch, TN 37013
(615) 831-3190 (H)
(615) 221-7272 (W)

Mobile Patriots
Milton Courington
1351 Barker Dr. East
Mobile, AL 36608
(205) 343-1166 (H)
(205) 431-3448 (W)

Atlanta Wheelchair Hawks
Patti Craig
Shepard Spinal Center
2020 Peachtree Road
Atlanta, GA 30309
(404) 350-2020 (W)

North Alabama Wheelers
Cindy Laney
19087 Coffman Road
Elkmont, AL 35620
(205) 232-7530 (H)
(205) 230-0035 (W)

West Division

Memphis River City Rollers
Kent Fiveash
5695 Green Valley
Memphis, TN 38135
(901) 383-8582 (H)
(901) 680-9032 (W)

New Orleans Rollin' Rino's
Rafael Ibarra
195 Cherokee Drive
Abita Springs, LA 70420
(504) 892-9724 (W)

Montgomery Mavericks
Laura Ward
P.O. Box 251123
Montgomery, AL 36105
(205) 278-3232 (H)

Jackson Rolling Tigers
John L. Dickerson
647 Queen Julianna Ln.
Jackson, MS 39209
(601) 922-3951 (H)

Jackson J-Wheelers
L.V. Thurman
3590 Albermarle B112
Jackson, MS 39213
(601) 366-9706 (W)
(601) 366-5282 (H)

Rome Rolling Romans
Charles Burke
16 Wheeler St.
Rome, GA 30161
(706) 235-0463 (H)

Conference Independent

Music City Lightning
William H. McCormack
1808 Rosebank Ave.
Nashville, TN 37216
(615) 226-1296 (H)

SOUTHERN CALIFORNIA

President
Roger Bogh
1017 Park Place
Coronado, CA 92118
(619) 524-1713 (W)
(619) 435-8792 (H)

Vice President
Mikel Bistany
5500 Irvine Center Dr.
Irvine, CA 92720
(714) 559-3243 (W)
(714) 262-0802 (H)

Secretary
Richard Huebsch
2231 E. Mercer Ln.
Phoenix, AZ 85028
(602) 971-7139 (H)

Treasurer
Ken McCulloch
206 S. Drexel Ave.
National City, CA 91950
(619) 694-2515 (W)
(619) 472-2261 (H)

Commissioner
Chuck Molnar
10757 Lemon Ave. #1903
Alta Loma, CA 91737
(909) 941-7021

Saddleback Gauchos
Brian Geier
30811 Calle Chueca
San Juan Capistrano, CA 92675
(714) 496-3349 (H)
(714) 582-4679 (W)

Cypress College Chariots
Bob Nadell
Dept. of PE
Cypress College
9200 Valley View
Cypress, CA 90630
(714) 761-0961 (W)

San Diego Olympians
Isaac Contraras
8009F Caminito de Pizza
San Diego, CA 92108
(619) 542-1367 (H)
(619) 524-1713 (W)

Loma Linda Rollercoasters
Lloyd Broyles
3148 Belvedere Drive
Riverside, CA 92507
(909) 799-6144 (W)
(909) 788-0940 (H)

Phoenix Sumaritan Suns
Kevin Rasmusson
1437 S. Revere

Mesa, AZ 85210
(602) 464-0391 (H)

Inland Empire Rolling Bear
Guy Perry
15131 San Jose Drive
Victorville, CA 92392
(619) 951-8250 (H)

Conference Independent

Irvine Valley College Lasers
Mikel Bistany
(see VP, above)

Casa Colina Condors
Greg A'Lurede
1194 Myra Ct.
Upland, CA 91786
(714) 982-1255 (H)

WISCONSIN

President
Carlos Mireles
24819 Adams Street
Kanasville, WI 53139
(414) 878-3662 (H)
(414) 636-4228 (W)

Vice President
Todd Palkowski
10564 W. Cortez Cir. #4
Franklin, WI 53132
(414) 529-5699 (H)
(414) 438-5622 (W)

Secretary/Treasurer
Dennis R. Gogin
1106 H Fleetfoot Dr.
Waukesha, WI 53186
(414) 544-96Z9 (H)
(414) 643-6501 (W)

Commissioner
Raymond A. Lorberter
2330 N. 62nd Street
Wauwatosa, WI 53213
(414) 257-2282 (H)

Mad City Bombers
Tim Valley
57 Walter St.
Madison, WI 53714
(608) 242-8628 (H)
(608) 233-1300 (W)

South Shore Breakers
Carlos Mireles
(see President, above)

Horizons
Jeff Liebzeit
1451 Planeview Dr.
Oshkosh, WI 54904
(414) 426-2629 (H)
(414) 589-2721 (W)

Milwaukee Spirit
Dennis R. Gogin
(See Sec/Treas., above)

Locating Assistive Technology and Other Information

The state information below was provided by Ohio's Technology Assistance Information Network (Ohio T.R.A.I.N.). Ohio T.R.A.I.N. is a federally funded project, awarded to the State of Ohio from the U.S. Department of Education, National Institute on Disability and Rehabilitation Research (N.I.D.R.R.). It is funded under the Tech Act which was passed in order to provide financial assistance to the states to support the development and implementation of a consumer responsive comprehensive state-wide program of technology related assistance for individuals of all ages with disabilities.

Each state has an office which provides information regarding assistive technology and other information to consumers. Assistive technology includes devices, comprehensive services and funding sources that accompany the provision of an appropriate piece of equipment for a person with a disability. These offices answer questions about assistive technology needs, including disseminating information about funding mechanisms, protective laws, state, local and private services, service providers, manufacturers, and products.

The consumer can call these offices to find out about manufacturers of sports and recreation equipment as well as a wealth of other information regarding other products and services which can assist in almost any area of life. These offices collect product catalogs, do database searching, and network among other agencies, offices, and companies, so that they bring to the consumer the most complete and up-to-date information. These offices also provide informational and training seminars and specialize in community outreach. In areas such as virtual reality, they are pushing the technology forward to create new applications of particular service to the disabled.

Assistive Technology Projects in the United States and Territories

Alabama:
Statewide Technology Access and Response (STAR) System for Alabamians with Disabilities

Alabama Department of Rehabilitation Services
2129 East South Blvd. P.O. Box 11586

Montgomery, AL 36111-0586
205/288-0240
Fax: 205/281-1973

Alaska:
Alaska Assistive Technology
Project
Department of Education
Div. of Vocational Rehabilitation
Assistive Technologies of Alaska
400 D Street, Suite 230
Anchorage, AK 99501
800/770-0138 (V/TT)
907/274-0138 (V/TT)
Fax: 907/274-0516

American Samoa:
American Samoa Assistive
Technology Service (ASATS)
Project
Division of Vocational Rehabili-
tation
Department of Human Resources
Pago Pago, American Samoa
96799
011/684-633-2336 (V)
011/684-633-1805 (V)
011/684-633-2393 (TT)
Fax: 011/684-633-2393

Arizona:
Arizona Technology Access
Program
(AzTAP)
Northern Arizona University
Arizona University Affiliated
Program
2600 North Wyatt Drive
Tucson, AZ 85712
602/324-3170 (V)
Fax: 602/324-3176

Arkansas:
Arkansas ICAN (Increasing

Capabilities Access Network)
Department of Education/Voca-
tional Education Division
Arkansas Rehabilitation Services
2201 Brookwood Drive, Ste. 117
Little Rock, AR 72202
800/828-2799 (V/TT) In state
only
501/666-8868 (V/TT)
Fax: 501/666-5319

California:
California Assistive Technology
System (CATS)
Department of Rehabilitation
Independent Living Division
830 K Street
Sacramento, CA 95814
916/327-3967 (V/TT)
Fax: 916/327-0914

Colorado:
Colorado Assistive Technology
Project: Developing Colo-
rado's Consumer Responsive
System
Rocky Mountain Resource and
Training Institute
6355 Ward Road, Suite 310
Arvada, CO 80004
303/420-2942 (V/TT)
Fax: 303/420-8675

Connecticut:
Connecticut Assistive Technol-
ogy Project
Connecticut Department of
Social Services
Bureau of Rehabilitation Services
10 Griffin Road North
Windsor, CT 06095
203/298-2042
Fax: 203/298-9590

Delaware:
Delaware Assistive Technology Initiative (DATI)
University of Delaware
Center for Applied Science and Engineering
A.I. Dupont Institute
1600 Rockland Road
P.O. Box 269
Wilmington, DE 19899
302/651-6830
Fax: 302/651-6793

District of Columbia:
District of Columbia Partnership for Assistive Technology (DCPAT)
District of Columbia Department of Human Services National Rehabilitation Hospital—Rehabilitation Engineering Department
801 Pennsylvania Avenue SE, Suite 210
Washington, DC 20003
202/546-9163 (V)
202/546-9168 (TT)
Fax: 202/546-9169

Florida:
Florida's Alliance for Assistive Services and Technology (FAAST)
Florida Department of Labor and Employment Security
Division of Vocational Rehabilitation
2002 Old St. Augustine Rd., Building A
Tallahassee, FL 32399-0696
904/488-8380
Fax: 904/488-8062

Tools for Life—Georgia Assistive Technology Program
Tools for Life
Georgia Department of Human Resources, Division of Rehabilitation Services
2 Peachtree Street NW, Suite 23-411
Atlanta, GA 30303-3166
800/497-8665 (V)
404/657-3082 (V)
404/657-3084 (V)
404/657-3085 (TT)
Fax: 404/657-3086

Guam:
Guam System for Assistive Technology (GSAT)
University of Guam
University Affiliated Program on Developmental Disabilities
UOG Station
Mangilao, GU 96923
671/734-9309
Fax: 671/734-5709

Hawaii:
Hawaii Assistive Technology System for Persons with Disabilities
Vocational Rehabilitation and Services for the Blind Division
1000 Bishop Street, Room 605
Honolulu, HI 96813
808/586-5375
Fax: 808/532-7120

Idaho:
Idaho Assistive Technology Project
Idaho Center on Developmental Disabilities
University of Idaho Professional Building

129 West Third Street
Moscow, ID 83844-4401
208/885-3559 (V/TT)
800/432-8324 (V/TT)—accessible to (208) & (509) area codes
Fax: 208/885-3628

Illinois:
Illinois Assistive Technology Project
Illinois Assistive Technology Project
110 Iles Park Place
Springfield, IL 62718
800/852-5110 (V/TT) In state only
217/522-9966 (TT)
Fax: 217/522-8067

Indiana:
Technology-Related Assistance for Individuals with Disabilities
ATTAIN
402 West Washington Street
P.O. Box 7083
Indianapolis, IN 46207-7083
800/545-7763 (V)
800/743-3333 (TT)
317/233-3394 (V/TT)
Fax: 317/232-6478

Iowa:
Technology Related Assistance for Individuals with Disabilities
Iowa Program for Assistive Technology
Room 217 UHS
University of Iowa
Iowa City, IA 52242
800/331-3027 (V/TT)
Fax: 319/356-8284

Kansas:
Assistive Technology for Kansans
University of Kansas
University Affiliated Program at Parsons Assistive Technology Center
2601 Gabriel
P.O. Box 738
Parsons, KS 67357
316/421-8367 (V)
316/421-0954 (TT/Fax)
Fax: 316/421-0954

Kentucky:
The Kentucky Assistive Technology Service (KATS) Network
Kentucky Department for the Blind
KATS Network Coordinating Center
427 Versailles Road
Frankfort, KY 40601
502/573-4665 (V/TT)
Fax: 502/573-3976
800/564-4665

Louisiana:
Louisiana Assistive Technology Access Network (LATAN)
Louisiana State Planning Council for Developmental Disabilities
P.O. Box 3455, Bin 14
1201 Capitol Access Road
Baton Rouge, LA 70821-3455
800/922-3425 (V)
800/256-1633 (TT)
504/342-2471 (V/TT)
Fax: 504/342-1970

Maine:
Maine Consumer Information and Technology Training Exchange (Maine CITE)
Maine Department of Education
Division of Special Services
State House Station #23
Augusta, ME 04333
207/621-3195 (V/TT)
Fax: 207/287-5900
207/621-3193

Maryland:
Maryland Technology Assistance Program (MTAP)
Governor's Office for Individuals with Disabilities
MD TAP
Box 10, One Market Center
300 W. Lexington Street
Baltimore, MD 21201
800/832-4827
800/TECH-TAP (V/TT)
410/333-4975
Fax: 410/889-5966

Massachusetts:
MATP Center
Massachusetts Commission for the Deaf and Hard of Hearing
600 Washington Street, Room 600
Boston, MA 02111
617/735-7820 (V)
617/735-7301 (TT)
800/848-8867 (V/TT)
Information and referral: 617/735-7153 (V)
Information and referral: 800/950-6287 (BBS) Tristate
617/267-5027 (BBS)
Fax: 617/735-6345

Michigan:
TECH 2000: Michigan's Assistive Technology Project
Michigan Rehabilitation Services
Community Development Division
P.O. Box 30010
Lansing, MI 48909
517/373-4058 (V)
517/373-4035 (TT)
Fax: 517/373-0565

Minnesota:
A System of Technology to Achieve Results (STAR)
State of Minnesota
Governor's Advisory Council on Technology for People with Disabilities
300 Centennial Building
658 Cedar Street
St. Paul, MN 55155
612/296-2771 (V)
612/296-9962 (TT)

Mississippi:
Project START—Success Through Assistive/Rehabilitative Technology
Department of Human Services
Office of Vocational Rehabilitation
P.O. Box 1000
Jackson, MS 39215
800/852-8328 (V/TT) In state only
601/987-4872 (V/TT)
Fax: 601/364-2349

Missouri:
Missouri Assistive Technology Project
Missouri Department of Labor & Industrial Relations

Governor's Committee on Employment of People with Disabilities
4731 South Cochise, Suite 114
Independence, MO 64055-6975
800/647-8557 (V)
800/647-8558 (TT)
816/373-5193 (V)
Fax: 816/373-9314

Montana:
MonTECH
Montana Department of Social and Rehabilitation Services
Rehabilitative Services Division
111 Sanders
P.O. Box 4210
Helena, MT 59604
800/732-0323 (V/TT)
406/243-5676 (V/TT)
406/243-2318
800/961-9610
(In MT and WY) (BBS-Rural Disability Information Network [RUDI])
Fax: 406/243-4730

Nebraska
Technology-Related Assistance Project
Nebraska Department of Education
Division of Vocational Rehabilitation
301 Centennial Mall South
P.O. Box 94987
Lincoln, NE 68509-4987
402/471-0734
402/471/3647 (V/TT)
Fax: 402/471-0117

New Hampshire:
Supporting People with Disabilities Through New Hampshire's Technology Partnership
Technology Partnership
Institute on Disability
10 Ferry Street, Suite 307, Unit 14
Concord, NH 03301
603/224-0630 (V/TT)
Fax: 603/862-0034

New Jersey:
Technology Assistive Resource Program
New Jersey Department of Labor
Division of Vocational Rehabilitation Services
CN 398, 135 East State Street, 1st Floor Trenton, NJ 08625
800/342-5832 (V) In state only
800/382-7765
800/DTARP-NJ (TT) In state only
Fax: 609/292-4616

New Mexico:
New Mexico Technology-Related Assistance Program (NMTAP)
State Department of Education
Division of Vocational Rehabilitation
435 Saint Michaels Drive, Building D
Santa Fe, NM 87505
800/866-2253
800/866-ABLE (V/TT)
800/659-4915 (TT)
505/827-3532 (V)
505/827-3587 (TT)
Fax: 505/827-3746

Nevada:
Assistive Technology Services, Advocacy, and Systems Change
Nevada Rehabilitation Division
Community-Based Services
711 South Stewart Street
Carson City, NV 89710
702/687-4452
Fax: 702/687-3292

New York:
Technology-Related Assistance of Individuals with Disabilities (TRAID)
New York State Office of Advocate for Persons with Disabilities
TRAID Project
One Empire State Plaza, Suite 1001
Albany, NY 12223-1150
800/522-4369 (V/TT) In state only
518/474-2825 (V)
518/473-4231 (TT)
Fax: 518/473-6005

North Carolina:
North Carolina Assistive Technology Project
North Carolina Assistive Technology Project
North Carolina Department of Human Resources
Division of Vocational Rehabilitation Services
1110 Navaho Drive, Suite 101
Raleigh, NC 27609
800/852-0042 (V/TT)
919/850-2787 (V/TT)
Fax: 919/850-2792

North Dakota:
Comprehensive Statewide Program of Technology-Related Assistance for Individuals with Disabilities
North Dakota Department of Human Services
Office of Vocational Rehabilitation
P.O. Box 743
Cavalier, ND 58220
701/265-4807 (V)
701/224-3975 (TT)
Fax: 701/265-3150

Northern Mariana Islands:
CNMI System of Technology-Related Assistance for Individuals with Disabilities
CNMI Governor's Developmental Disabilities Council
Commonwealth of Northern Mariana Islands
P.O. Box 2565
Capitol Hill
Saipan, MP 96950
670/322-3015 (V)
670/322-3014 (V/TT)
Fax: 670/322-4168

Ohio:
Ohio Project on Technology-Related Assistance for Individuals with Disabilities (Ohio T.R.A.I.N.—Tech Act Project)
Ohio T.R.A.I.N.
Ohio Super Computer Center
1224 Kinnear Rd.
Columbus, Ohio 43212
614/292-2426 (V/TT)
800/784-3425 (V/TT) In state only
Fax: 614/292-5866

Oklahoma:
Oklahoma Assistive Technology Program
Oklahoma Department of Rehabilitation
P.O. Box 36659
Oklahoma City, OK 73136
405/424-4311, ext. 2722 (V)
405/424-4311, ext. 2825 (TT)
Fax: 405/427-3027

Oregon:
Technology Access for Life Needs
Department of Human Resources
Vocational Rehabilitation Division—TALN
Chemeketa Community College
4000 Lancaster Drive NE
P.O. Box 14007
Salem, OR 97309-7070
800/677-7512 In state only
Fax: 503/399-6978

Pennsylvania:
Pennsylvania's Technology
Temple University
Institute on Disabilities/UAP
Ritter Annex, Room 433
Philadelphia, PA 19122
800/204-PIAT
215/204-1356 (V/TT)
Fax: 215/204-6336

Puerto Rico:
Puerto Rico Assistive Technology Program for Individuals with Disabilities
UPR-RCM-CPRS
Department of Communication Disorders
Puerto Rico Assistive Technology Program (PRATP)
Box 365067

San Juan, PR 00936-5067
800/496-6035 (U.S.)
800/981-6033 (P.R.)
809/758-2525 ext. 4402, 4406, 4413, 4412
Fax: 809/759-3645

Rhode Island:
Rhode Island Assistive Technology Access Partnership (ATAP)
Rhode Island Department of Human Services
Office of Rehabilitation Services
40 Fountain Street
Providence, RI 02903-1898
401/421-7005 (V)
401/421-7016 (TT)
Fax: 401/421-9259

South Carolina:
South Carolina Assistive Technology Program
South Carolina Vocational Rehabilitation Department
P.O. Box 15
1410-C Boston Avenue
West Columbia, SC 29171-0015
800/922-1107 (V/TT) Access Technology Referral Line
803/822-5404 (V/TT)

South Dakota:
DakotaLink
State of South Dakota Department of Human Services/Division of Rehabilitation
East Highway 34, Hillsview Plaza
c/o 500 East Capitol
Pierre, SD 57501-5070
800/645-0673 (V/TT)
605/394-1876
Fax: 605/394-5315

Tennessee:
Tennessee Technology Access Project
Department of Mental Health and Mental Retardation
Tennessee Technology Access
Gateway Plaza—Eleventh Floor
710 James Robertson Parkway
Nashville, TN 37243-0381
800/732-5059 In state only
Fax: 615/741-0770

Texas:
Texas Assistive Technology Partnership Project
Texas Consortium for Developmental Disabilities AUAP
The University of Texas at Austin
Department of Special Education, EDB
Room 306
Austin, TX 78712-1290
800/828-7839 (V/TT) In state only
512/471-7621 (V)
Fax: 512/471-7549

Utah:
Utah Assistive Technology Program (UATP)
Utah State University
Utah Center for Assistive Technology (UCAT)
Center for Persons with Disabilities, UMC 6800
Logan, UT 84322-6855
801/797-2153 (V)
801/797-2096 (TT);
Fax: 801/797-2355

Vermont:
Assistive Technology Development Grant

Vermont Assistive Technology Project
Department of Aging and Disabilities
103 South Main Street
Waterbury, VT 05676
800/639-1522 (V/TT) In state only
Fax: 802/241-3052

Technical Assistance Contract
RESNA
1700 N. Moore Street, Suite 1540
Arlington, VA 22209-1903
703/524-6686
Fax: 703/524-6630

Virginia:
Virginia Assistive Technology
Department of Rehabilitative Services
VATS
8004 Franklin Farms Drive
Richmond, VA 23288-0300
800/435-8490 (V/TT) In state only
800/238-7955 (BBS)
Fax: 804/662-9478

Washington:
Washington Assistive Technology Project
Division of Vocational Rehabilitation
Department of Social and Health Services
University of Washington Affiliated Programs
Washington Department of Services for the Blind
P. O. Box 45340
Olympia, WA 98504-5340
206/438-8051
Fax: 206/438-8007

Wisconsin:
Technology-Related Assistance for Individuals with Disabilities: WisTech
Wisconsin Department of Health and Social Services
Division of Vocational Rehabilitation
P.O. Box 7852
Madison, WI 53707-7852
608/266-1281
Fax: 608/267-3657

West Virginia:
West Virginia Assistive Technology System (WVATS)
West Virginia Division of Rehabilitation Services
Capitol Complex

Charleston, WV 25305-0890
800/841-8436 (V/TT) In state only
304/293-4692 (V/TT)
Fax: 304/766-4671

Wyoming:
Wyoming's New Options in Technology (WYNOT)
State of Wyoming Department of Employment
Wyoming Division of Vocational Rehabilitation
1100 Herschler Building
Cheyenne, WY 82002
307/777-7450 (V)
800/877-9965 (TT)
Fax: 307/777-5939

Americans with Disabilities Act (ADA) and Recreation

What Is the ADA?

To the more than 43 million (some estimate 49 million) citizens with disabilities, the Americans with Disabilities Act (ADA) is an unprecedented opportunity to eliminate barriers to independence and productivity. The ADA is modeled after the Civil Rights Act of 1964 and Title V of the Rehabilitation Act of 1973. The purpose of the ADA is to extend to people with disabilities civil rights similar to those previously made available to citizens on the basis of race, color, sex, national origin, and religion in the Civil Rights Act of 1964. The ADA prohibits discrimination on the basis of disability in:

- employment
- services rendered by state and local governments
- places of public accommodation
- transportation and telecommunications.

Services rendered by state and local government and places of public accommodation are particularly important to recreation services. This covers city and state parks, schools, state-funded colleges, and such facilities as arenas and stadiums. National Parks are covered by the 1981 Uniform Accessibility Standards. Citizens—children and adults alike—may not know they have rights in all of these areas, but they do. Under the ADA, disabled children are entitled to a proper adapted physical education in their public school. Yet the vast majority of disabled children do not participate in such programs. The ADA mandates that properly adapted fitness programs must become more widely available in both the community and rehabilitation settings to enable people to be more independent and physically fit. These are civil rights.

Local Parks and Playgrounds

Cities, towns, and villages have the responsibility of modifying their facilities to meet ADA standards. This affects such services as city parks and playgrounds. These facilities serve both young people and adults, with services including both playgrounds for the young and areas to work out, swim, or enjoy other fitness, recreation, and sport activities enjoyed by the rest of the community. Even though a city may face severe budget restraints, it cannot simply eliminate or ignore the mandate of the ADA. The courts have consistently upheld the rights of disabled citizens to enjoy facilities in their communities. But this is not an unlimited right. For example, not every park has to be adapted. The modifications can take place over time, providing the government entity can show it is taking steps. The ADA requires that the parks and playgrounds, when viewed in their entirety within a community, are accessible to individuals with disabilities.

The National League of Cities published this checklist to evaluate the park or recreational property:

1. How do people with disabilities learn about your recreational programs and facilities?
2. Are there sufficient numbers of accessible parking spaces for people with disabilities at each site?
3. Can people with disabilities get from the parking lot to accessible facilities unassisted?
4. Are ground surfaces for accessible areas stable, firm and slip resistant?
5. Has playground equipment been adapted for children with disabilities?
6. Have other recreational areas and equipment been adapted for people with disabilities (swimming pools, golf carts, boat landings)?
7. Are trails marked for use by people with visual impairments?
8. Are public programs such as wildflower walks, and information centers, accessible to people with hearing impairments?
9. Are public buildings including restrooms, drinking fountains, and picnic tables accessible to people using wheelchairs?

("Recreation Facilities Top List of ADA Challenges for Cities," Kathryn S. McCarthy and Dianne C. Lipsey. *Nation's Cities Weekly*; May 16, 1994)

Federal Contacts

If you need to contact the federal office regarding ADA compliance, you can use the following numbers:

For enforcement of provisions dealing with public accommodations:

Civil Rights Division	202/514-0301
Office of the ADA	202/514-0383 (TDD)
U.S. Department of Justice	

For enforcement of transportation provisions, you should contact the Department of Transportation   202/366-9305
202/514-0383 (TDD)

State Contacts

If you need to contact your state office regarding an ADA violation or compliance issue in your state, you can use the following numbers:*

ALABAMA:
205/242-7983
ALASKA:
907/465-2814
ARIZONA:
602/542-6276
ARKANSAS:
501/324-9106
CALIFORNIA:
916/327-0437
COLORADO:
303/368-4100
CONNECTICUT:
203/298-2027
DELAWARE:
302/577-2850
FLORIDA:
904/488-8062

GEORGIA:
404/657-7313
HAWAII:
808/586-5366
IDAHO:
208/334-2873
ILLINOIS:
217/785-0234
INDIANA:
317/232-7770
IOWA:
515/281-4026
KANSAS:
913/296-3011
KENTUCKY:
502/564-7530
LOUISIANA:
504/342-7000

* These phone numbers were compiled by Mary Ann Farrell and originated in the Knight-Ridder Tribune News Service.

Sports, Everyone!

MAINE:
207/624-5308
MARYLAND:
410/333-2263
MASSACHUSETTS:
617/727-7440
MICHIGAN:
517/373-3391
MINNESOTA:
612/296-5616
MISSISSIPPI:
601/359-3511
MISSOURI:
314/751-2600
MONTANA:
406/444-2590
NEBRASKA:
402/471-4285
NEVADA:
702/687-4440
NEW HAMPSHIRE:
603/271-2773
NEW JERSEY:
609/292-7299
NEW MEXICO:
505/827-3538
NEW YORK:
518/474-2714
NORTH DAKOTA:
701/224-3991
OHIO:
614/438-1391

OKLAHOMA:
405/424-4311
OREGON:
503/378-3142
PENNSYLVANIA:
717/787-9353
RHODE ISLAND:
401/277-3731
SOUTH CAROLINA:
803/253-6336
SOUTH DAKOTA:
605/773-4918
TENNESSEE:
615/741-6380
TEXAS:
512/483-4422
UTAH:
801/538-7530
VERMONT:
802/828-3322
VIRGINIA:
804/662-7069
WASHINGTON:
206/438-3168
WEST VIRGINIA:
304/766-4600
WISCONSIN:
608/266-5378
WYOMING:
307/777-7191

Architectural Guidelines

To request ADA Accessibility Guidelines (ADAAG) required under Title III (public accommodations) and technical assistance on architectural, transportation, and communications accessibility issues, please call:

Architectural and Transportation Barriers Compliance Board (called the Access Board), 800/USA-ABLE; 800/USA-ABLE (TDD)

Index of Associations, Camps, and Schools

Index of Sports and Activities

The sports and activities listed are followed by organizations and institutions that offer or promote them, and the pages numbers on which those organizations and institutions are found.

Fitness
Southern Illinois University at
Carbondale, 108
Temple University, 110

**Flag Football (*see also* Football,
Wheelchair Football)**
American Athletic Association
for the Deaf (AAAD), 38

Flying (*see also* Soaring)
Challenge Air for Kids and
Friends, 49
International Wheelchair Avia-
tors, 63

Football
Edinboro University of Pennsyl-
vania, 102
Gallaudet University, 103
Ohio State University, 111

**Freshwater Fishing (*see also*
Deep Sea Fishing, Fishing)**
Casa Colina/Work It Out Pro-
gram, 49

General Recreation
Amputees in Motion (AIM), 43
Ball State University, 101
Ohio State University, 111
Parks & Recreation Department,
Santa Barbara, CA, 80
Temple University, 110

General Sports
Boy Scouts of America, 45
Girl Scouts of the USA, 62

Goalball
U.S. Association for Blind Athletes (USABA), 88

Golf
American Athletic Association
for the Deaf (AAAD), 38
Amputees in Motion (AIM), 43
National Amputee Golf Associa-
tion (NAGA), 64
Special Olympics International,
82
United States Blind Golfers, 93

Gymnastics
Special Olympics International,
82

Handball. *See* Team Handball

Hang Gliding
University of Wisconsin at
Whitewater, 117

Hayrides
National Sports Center for the
Disabled, 69

Hiking (*see also* Backpacking)
Breckenridge Outdoor Education
Center Activity, 46
Cooperative Wilderness Handi-
capped Outdoor Group
(C.W. Hog), 50
National Sports Center for the
Disabled, 69

**Hockey. *See* Ice Hockey; Sledge
Hockey**

Horseback Riding
Amputees in Motion (AIM), 43
ASPIRE (Association of Special
People Inspired to Riding), 44
National Library Service for the
Blind and Physically Handi-
capped, 68

Appendix

Getting Involved in Recreation Planner

by John A. Nesbitt, Ed.D.
Special Recreation, Inc.

This planner helps you get involved in the recreation activities you most enjoy and will benefit you. It is designed to be interactive. Hopefully the exercises will help you learn more about yourself and focus your priorities.

First you take inventory of the recreation you enjoy using the **"Recreation I Most Enjoy"** checklist.

Next you put your budget together using **Section II,** seeing what you spent this year and how much you expect to spend next year.

Next you analyze the barriers to recreation using a series of checklists in **Section III, "Overcoming Personal and Community Barriers."** Using these checklists, you can assess where the barriers are and how you can work to overcome them.

Section IV gives you a list of options to open your mind to activities and opportunities. You should supplement this with your own list of activities.

Section V helps you examine the satisfaction and benefits you derive from your recreation pursuits. Choose an activity from the list from section IV or from you own list. Assess why you do it and what you get from it.

Section VI helps you evaluate your skill levels for your chosen activities.

Section VII helps you identify what events you have participated in in your community.

Section VIII pulls it all together. Make your calendar with your selected activities on the basis of budget, barriers, benefits, and skills. Now, enjoy your year!

I. THE RECREATION I MOST ENJOY

Check the recreation activities you most enjoy. Fill in others which do not appear on this checklist. You may think of whole new categories.

Creative
- ❑ Arts and Crafts, creation
- ❑ Arts and Crafts, viewing
- ❑ Other_____

Culture
- ❑ Concert hall, music, drama
- ❑ Other_____

Entertainment
- ❑ Movies
- ❑ Radio
- ❑ Television
- ❑ Videos
- ❑ Other_____

Home
- ❑ Loafing, resting
- ❑ Gardening
- ❑ Fixup
- ❑ Entertaining
- ❑ Special foods
- ❑ Other_____

Social
- ❑ Family
- ❑ Friends
- ❑ Clubs and Groups
- ❑ Politics
- ❑ Other_____

Music
- ❑ Music, listening
- ❑ Music, playing and singing
- ❑ Other_____

Outdoor Recreation
- ❑ Camping
- ❑ Fishing
- ❑ Hunting
- ❑ Other_____

Sports
- ❑ Individual
- ❑ Team
- ❑ Indoor
- ❑ Outdoor

Reading
- ❑ Books
- ❑ Papers
- ❑ Magazines

Serving Others
- ❑ Leading, coaching, teaching
- ❑ Volunteering, community service
- ❑ Other_____

Special Interests
- ❑ Religion
- ❑ Cultural or Ethnic
- ❑ Other_____

Travel
- ❑ In the State
- ❑ In the Region
- ❑ Nationwide
- ❑ Foreign

II. PUTTING TOGETHER YOUR RECREATION BUDGET

You should determine your cost according to the following schedule: monthly, annual, and projection for next year.

	Monthly $ Cost	Annual $ Cost	Next Year $ Cost
	(DE-Decrease IN-Increase SA-Same)		
Books and Subscriptions:			
Electronics:			
Instructional Videos:			
Fees (admissions, dues, licenses, memberships, services):			
Food and related items:			
Hobby (costs, equipment, materials, supplies, tools, etc.):			
Music and Art:			
Pets:			
Sports (clothing, equipment, supplies, travel):			
Travel and Vacation (fares, food, services, etc.):			
Other:			
Other:			
Other:			

III. OVERCOMING COMMUNITY AND PERSONAL BARRIERS TO RECREATION

To enjoy recreation, you may need to overcome community and personal barriers. You may need to find facilities which are ADA compliant. You may need to educate yourself about adaptive/assistive equipment and means for funding. You may need to train yourself in certain skills and join certain groups in your region in order to participate in team and group activities. The first step is to identify the barriers and the second step is to work on a strategy to overcome them. Some barriers will be more in your control than others.

	No Barrier	Minor	Moderate	Major	Worst Barrier
(Check Box)					
Cost Barriers					
Instruction					
Equipment					
Materials					
Admission, fees, membership					
Transportation					
Personal Skill and Motivation Level					
Lack of training					
Lack of instructional material					
Lack of desire or motivation					
Lack of friend or companion to recreate with					
Lack of energy					

	No Barrier	Minor	Moderate	Major	Worst Barrier
Lack of self-esteem to join, enter					
Other:					
Resources					
Lack of sources of information, referral, networking					
Lack of national, state, or local organization to join					
Lack of national support for program development					
Transportation					
Transportation to and from					
Other:					
Program-Service Deficiencies					
Lack of enough people to allow an activity					
Lack of program or service					
Lack of trained staff, leaders, teachers					

	No Bar-rier	Minor	Moder-ate	Major	Worst Barrier
Lack of adapted or modified equipment					
Lack of adapted or modified facility					
Lack of organized consumer group					
Other:					
Overall Barriers					
Architectural barriers to access					
Attitudinal barriers of staff					
Attitudinal barriers of public					

Checklist of Strategies to Overcome Barriers

Look over these strategies asking the following questions. The answers may help you find ways to overcome the barriers you have identified.

Ask the following PLANNING questions:
- Who needs the recreation activity? Age? How many?
- Why is the recreation needed?
- What recreation activities are needed?
- When (days, times) and where (location) is the recreation needed?
- How do you see the recreation activity or program being provided?
- What friends, other parents, other groups, etc., support your request?

- What other support or assistance (costs, volunteers, transportation) is needed?

Ask the following STRATEGY questions:
- What do I want?
- Direct services?
- Indirect or support services?
- Who should I contact? (public/government; voluntary, commercial)
- What resources can I use?

IV. CHECKLIST OF RECREATION OPTIONS

What's on your schedule for recreation today, this week, this month?

- ☐ **Act,** creative drama, community theater, storytelling
- ☐ **Advocate,** for better education, government, recreation or wilderness
- ☐ **Animals,** keep or care of pets, animal protection society, animal husbandry
- ☐ **Art,** draw, paint, sculpt, display art, join an art group
- ☐ **Business,** make a product, provide a service, sell an item or line
- ☐ **Camping,** day, overnight, resident, mountaineering, RVehicle, wilderness
- ☐ **Clubs,** advocacy, civic, consumer, fraternal, hobby, self-help, social
- ☐ **Collecting,** antiques, books, collectibles, coins, memorabilia, stamps
- ☐ **Computer,** play computer games, join an online system, surf the Internet
- ☐ **Cooking,** specialties, exchange cooking group, learn to cook, teach cooking
- ☐ **Crafts,** cloth, gems, glass, paper, plastic, metal, modeling, toys, wood
- ☐ **Current Events,** write a letter to an editor, attend a public meeting
- ☐ **Cycling,** one wheel, two wheel, three wheel, tandem, racing, touring
- ☐ **Dance,** folk dancing, latest dance, social dancing, square dancing
- ☐ **Drama,** attend a movie, a play, join a drama group
- ☐ **Driving,** car, RV-camper, special vehicle, car clubs, competitive driving
- ☐ **Education,** correspondence course, college course, TV course, for fun or profit
- ☐ **Ethnic,** arts, customs, dress, games, history, songs, sports, stories, trades
- ☐ **Family,** anniversaries, birthdays, fun, genealogy, projects, reunions, travel
- ☐ **Fishing,** lake, river, stream, saltwater, pole fishing, casting, trolling
- ☐ **Fitness/Wellness,** every day—aerobics, limbering, walking
- ☐ **Food,** eat recreationally (eat less but enjoy it more)
- ☐ **Games,** play old games, learn new games, make games, collect games, tournaments
- ☐ **Garden,** tend to indoor/outdoor garden, plants, attend a garden show, exhibit
- ☐ **Hobbies,** display your hobby, start a new hobby, teach someone your hobby

- **Home**, check for hazards, fix something, install a convenience, redecorate
- **Hunting**, archery, rifle and shotgun hunting, spear hunting
- **Leading**, playground or room leader, recreation leader, youth leader, coach
- **Letters/Tapes/Computer E-mail**, to friends, relatives, pen-pals, tape exchange clubs
- **Museums**, art, ethnic, history, science, natural history, or create a museum
- **Music**, listen to the radio, play stereo or CD player, attend a concert
- **Nature Study**, birdwatch, explore caves, study flora and fauna
- **Outdoor Recreation,** backpack, climb, join an outdoor club
- **Organize**, a club, a study group, a community group, a service group, a project
- **Photography**, black and white, color, movies, videotaping, display
- **Play an Instrument**, horn, piano, percussion, stringed instrument, electronic instruments
- **Radio and TV**, radio listening, TV, ham radio, closed-circuit television
- **Read,** fiction, non-fiction, poetry, plays, read for others, join a group
- **Relaxation**, contemplation, reflection, meditation, stress reduction
- **Running,** jogging, jogging events, racing events, join a running group, marathons
- **Singing**, join a choir or singing group, attend a singing program, singalong
- **Social Recreation**, anniversaries, birthdays, parties, coffees, dinners
- **Speaking**, join a speakers' group, give school or public talks, debate
- **Special Event**, national holiday, patriotic observance, religious activity
- **Skilled Trades,** carpentry, masonry, mechanics, repair for service or profit
- **Sports,** individual, teams, seasonal, indoor, outdoor, tournaments, camps, training
- **Teach,** children, youngsters, adults, students, community groups
- **Touring**, plan a trip, take a trip, share trip slides and memorabilia
- **Voluntary Service**, civic group, center, community, hospital, neighborhood
- **Walk,** hike, orienteer, racewalk, stroll
- **Water Recreation**, boat, canoe, dive, sail, SCUBA, surf, swim
- **Write,** anecdote, autobiography, letter, newsletter, poem, short story

V. RECREATION BENEFITS, JOYS, OUTCOMES, SATISFACTION

What do you get from your recreation? Are you going through the motions of an activity, or participating with the result nothing more than "killing time"? Ask yourself what satisfactions you are getting from which recreation.

For each of your recreation pursuits identified in the preceding options list, rate the experience by placing a letter which best reflects the type of satisfaction you are deriving from the activity. This inventory will help you focus on the pursuits most fulfilling to you.

N=Never   **S**=Sometimes   **U**=Usually   **A**=Always

Recreation Pursuit:_____

___Amusement
___Achievement
        ___personal fulfillment
        ___highest potential
___Aesthetic fulfillment
___Creative fulfillment
___Diversion
___Education for recreation
        ___recreation philosophy and values
        ___recreation skills and competencies
        ___recreation resources
        ___recreation lifestyle
___Emotional
        ___release, reduction of stress and tension
        ___mental fitness
___Enjoyment
___Fun
___New experience
___Physical
        ___development
        ___maintenance
        ___stimulation
___Pleasure
___Relaxation
___Self-Expression
___Social

      ___relationships

      ___support

___Therapeutic benefits

      ___escape from physical pain or mental anguish

      ___relief from boredom, isolation, regimentation

      ___therapy for emotional, mental, physical, or social problems

      ___enhancement of affective-emotional, cognitive-mental, physical and/or social functioning

___Wellness

      ___mental

      ___physical

VI. RECREATION SKILLS AND EXPERIENCE

The more skill and experience you have in a particular recreation pursuit, the more likely it is that you will greatly enjoy the pursuit.

Where do you have the most skills and experience and where do you need or want to improve?

To review your skills, take your list of pursuits. Put M next to where you are a master (aim for 3). Write I for where you have intermediate skills (aim for 5). And write N next to your novice pursuits (aim for 7). Once you have done this, you will have a clearer picture of where your skills take you, where you want to be, and where you want to put your efforts. This will help you draw up your own recreational calendar.

VII. RECREATION EVENTS

Are you getting out and about in your community? These events offer ways of keeping up with family and friends, knowing what is going on in your community, getting in touch with recreational, educational, and vocational opportunities.

Check the events that you attended/participated in over the last year and which you plan to attend again.

I attended this year:	I will attend next year:
❑ Anniversaries	❑
❑ Auctions	❑
❑ Birthdays	❑
❑ Carnivals	❑
❑ Commemorations	❑
❑ Competitions	❑
❑ Contests	❑
❑ Days	❑
❑ Festivals	❑
❑ Games	❑
❑ Jubilees	❑
❑ Months	❑
❑ Meetings	❑
❑ Readings	❑
❑ Theme Days, Events	❑
❑ Tournaments	❑
❑ Weeks	❑

VIII. MAKE YOUR CALENDAR

Plan ahead...monthly, seasonally, annually

Activity	Autumn SeptOctNov	Winter DecJanFeb	Spring MarAprMay	Summer JunJulAug
Advocate				
Act				
Animals				
Art				
Business				
Camping				
Clubs				
Collecting				
Computer				
Cooking				
Crafts				
Current Events				
Cycling				
Dance				
Drama				
Driving				
Education				
Ethnic				
Family				
Fishing				

Sports, Everyone!

Activity	Autumn SeptOctNov	Winter DecJanFeb	Spring MarAprMay	Summer JunJulAug
Fitness/Well-ness				
Food				
Games				
Garden				
Hobbies				
Home				
Hunting				
Leading				
Museums				
Music				
Nature				
Outdoor Recre-ation				
Organize, a club				
Photography				
Play an Instru-ment				
Radio and TV				
Read				
Relaxation				
Running				
Singing				
Social Recre-ation				

Activity	Autumn SeptOctNov	Winter DecJanFeb	Spring MarAprMay	Summer JunJulAug
Speaking				
Special Event				
Skilled Trades				
Sports				
Teach				
Touring				
Voluntary Service				
Walk				
Water Recreation				
Write				

The Credo of Special Recreation for People with Disabilities

We believe that every person
regardless of disability, illness, or injury
has the right...

• To achieve her or his highest potential for the pursuit of happiness and personal fulfillment through recreation;

• To equal opportunity in recreation, exercising this basic, democratic, human, and civil right without prejudice and at parity with society at large;

• To live a recreation lifestyle in the mainstream of society from infancy through childhood and adolescence, to adulthood, and as a senior;

• To exercise all consumers prerogatives and the range of choices available to the public based on individual needs, rights, interests, and aspirations;

• To call on the goodwill of the community and its resources to provide equal recreation opportunity through special recreation programs, services and staffing, and through creation advising/counseling and creation education for people with disabilities;

• To access to all recreation pursuits through adaptation, modification, and adjustment that overcome architectural, equipment, facility and transportation barriers;

• To receive the personal benefits of recreation including the affective, cognitive, development, emotional, health, physical, social, spiritual, and therapeutic benefits of recreation experience;

• To receive the therapeutic benefits of professional recreational therapies including activity, animal, aquatics, arts, child health, dance, drama, equestrian, horticulture, humor, music, photography, play, poetry/writing, recreation, reading, and sports; and

• To receive the rehabilitative benefits of recreation in services including activity, counseling, corrections, development, education and special education, employment and sheltered employment, home care, hospital care, institutional care, medical care, mental health, nursing care, occupational therapy, physical education, physical medicine and rehabilitation, physical therapy, psychotherapy, recreation service, residential care, social service, speech and hearing therapy, vocational rehabilitation, volunteer service, and wellness service.

We believe that every person
regardless of disability, illness, or injury
has the responsibility...

• To strive to achieve his or her highest potential for the pursuit of happiness, personal fulfillment, and quality of life in and through recreation; and

• To direct her or his recreation lifestyle by pursuing the aesthetic, cognitive, developmental, emotional, health, physical, social spiritual and therapeutic benefits of recreation.